Understanding Breast Cancer G

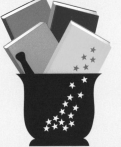

be well
informed

@ your library®

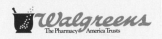
ALA American Library Association   Walgreens The Pharmacy America Trusts

This book was received through a grant from
Walgreens and the American Library Association.

Understanding Health and Sickness Series
Miriam Bloom, Ph.D.
General Editor

Understanding Breast Cancer Genetics

Barbara T. Zimmerman, Ph.D.

University Press of Mississippi
Jackson

www.upress.state.ms.us

The University Press of Mississippi is a member of the Association of American University Presses.

Illustrations by Alan Estridge

11 10 09 08 07 06 05 04 03 4 3 2 1
∞
Library of Congress Cataloging-in-Publication Data
Zimmerman, Barbara T.
    Understanding breast cancer genetics / Barbara T. Zimmerman.
        p. ; cm. — (Understanding health and sickness series)
Includes bibliographical references and index.
    ISBN 1-57806-578-X (cloth : alk. paper) — ISBN 1-57806-579-8
(paper : alk. paper)
        1. Breast—Cancer—Genetic aspects. 2. Breast—Cancer—Popular works.

    [DNLM: 1. Breast Neoplasms—genetics—Popular Works. WP 870 Z72u
2003] I. Title. II. Series.
    RC280.B8Z55 2003
    616.99′449042—dc21   2003007160

British Library Cataloging-in-Publication Data available

Contents

Acknowledgments

This book could not have been written without the help and support of many people. I am deeply indebted to my editor, Miriam Bloom, Ph.D. for her advice and understanding. I am especially grateful to Catherine Klein, M.D. (Hereditary Cancer Clinic, VA Medical Center, and Division of Medical Oncology, University of Colorado Health Sciences Center, Denver, CO) for critically reviewing the first draft of the manuscript and for her valuable suggestions. Several breast cancer specialists took time to discuss their areas of expertise with me. Andrew Kraft, M.D. (Chair, Division of Medical Oncology, University of Colorado Health Sciences Center) reviewed current diagnostic and treatment protocols. Anthony Elias, M.D. (Director, Clinical Breast Cancer Program, University of Colorado Hospital), discussed DNA microarray technology and its potential application to the diagnosis and treatment of breast cancer. Jeffrey Levy, M.D. (Chair, Department of Radiology, Rose Medical Center, Denver) discussed the controversies surrounding mammography and guided me to the most current sources of information. Jennifer Richer, Ph.D., an associate of Dr. Kathryn Horwitz (Division of Endocrinology, Metabolism, and Diabetes, University of Colorado Health Sciences Center), reviewed their current research on the interactions between progesterone and estrogen receptors in breast cancer cells. Lisen Axell, M.S. (Division of Cancer Prevention and Control, University of Colorado Health Sciences Center), gave me the perspective of a genetics counselor on the risks faced by patients with mutations in BRCA1 and BRCA2 genes. The late Carolyn Jaffe presented the perspective of a hospice nurse. Rena Bloom, N.D. and Jacob Schor, N.D. (Denver Naturopathic Clinic) shared their experiences as naturopathic physicians who advocate co-treatments with conventional therapies for breast cancer. Several close friends who are breast cancer patients and survivors shared their experiences with me, enabling me to add a human voice to the manuscript. My husband, Steven L. Zimmerman, and my daughter, Robin L. Hanssen, read the manuscript from the perspective of educated but non-medical readers and offered many helpful suggestions. I am forever grateful to my late father, Dr. Abraham Prostkoff, for encouraging my interest in biomedical research and in medicine, and I would like to thank my mother, Edith R. Prostkoff, for her enthusiastic support of this project and all my endeavors.

Introduction

Although an American woman is more likely to die of heart disease or of lung cancer, a diagnosis of breast cancer is the medical pronouncement she is most likely to fear. A woman often equates the breast with her femininity, sexuality, and psyche, and may fear possible disfigurement even more than death. This very fear may cause her to avoid simple screening procedures such as mammograms or self-examinations. She may delay seeking medical advice even after finding a lump. Consequences of this avoidance may be the difference between life and death.

While most women who develop breast cancer have no family history of the disease, some may have a number of close relatives who also had breast cancer or even died from it. Healthy young women with strong family histories of breast cancer often fear that they are doomed to develop the disease. They also fear passing a "bad" gene to their children. Tests have been developed to screen for such genes, but many women fear the implications of such tests. What are the consequences of learning that you carry such a gene? How will it affect your chances of obtaining employment or insurance? How do you live with the knowledge that you are at increased risk of developing breast cancer at a young age and that you may possibly die from the disease? Should you undergo radical prophylactic surgery to possibly save your life?

Recent advances in the Human Genome Project offer promises of cures for many genetically based diseases. Breakthroughs in molecular biology techniques now allow us to understand diseases such as cancer at their most basic level—the gene. Although only a small fraction of breast cancers are truly inherited, we know that damage to genes is involved in all cancers. In this context, breast cancer is a genetic disease and perhaps will eventually be cured by genetic manipulation.

Not long ago, breast cancer was not discussed in public. It was considered to be a private, sensitive issue generating feelings of embarrassment and even shame. Unfortunate victims often

underwent disfiguring radical mastectomies, only to die several
years later from recurring disease. Their survivors knew of their suf-
fering, but could only hope they wouldn't suffer the same fate.

Times have changed. We live in an exciting era of new technolog-
ical advances in medicine. Diagnostic tests can detect cancers at
early, more curable stages. Surgical treatments offer smaller incisions
and post-operative reconstruction. Today, breast cancer is a topic
that often makes headlines, especially when the patient is a celebrity.
Prominent women including Betty Ford, Happy Rockefeller, Shirley
Temple Black, former Colorado first lady Dottie Lamm, and Olivia
Newton-John have boldly announced their diseases to the world,
sharing their fear and anger and pain as well as their hope and deter-
mination to survive. They have encouraged women to be screened
regularly to detect early tumors that could be treated. They have
made women realize that breast cancer can happen to anyone and
that it is not a reason for shame. Survivors and their families continue to rally Congress for increased funding for breast cancer
research and have created organizations such as the Susan G. Komen
Foundation to raise funds for research and to provide breast cancer
education. Participation in the Komen Foundation's "Race for the
Cure" increases each year: In Denver, 1,600 participated in 1997,
27,000 in 1998, and nearly 53,000 in 2000! Women everywhere
wear distinctive pink ribbons announcing that they care about those
with breast cancer. Television anchors encourage women to do
monthly self-examinations and to go for mammograms.

And yet, the incidence of breast cancer is rising. An American
woman today has a one in eight chance of contracting the disease in
her lifetime, and over 40,000 still die of the disease. No one is
immune from breast cancer—not even men. It is still not understood why some individuals contract breast cancer and others do
not. Even women who have inherited mutations in the known susceptibility genes for breast cancer, BRCA1 and BRCA2, do not necessarily develop the disease. It must be that environment plays a role
in the expression of those genes.

This book has been written to help general readers understand
the genetic bases of both sporadic and inherited breast cancers. It is

most timely in this era of progress in the Human Genome Project and attempts at correcting genetic defects by gene therapy. I begin this book with a discussion of who gets breast cancer, breaking down patients by age of onset, ethnicity, sex, and implications for survival. Differences between sporadic and inherited breast cancers are considered. Chapter 2 introduces the general biology of cancer, and specifically breast cancer. The biology of different types of breast cancer is described with emphasis on how sporadic versus inherited forms arise and how the location of tumors can affect the outcome. In chapter 3, the concept of genes is introduced: what they are and what role they play in normal and cancerous cells. Chapter 4 focuses on the role of BRCA1, BRCA2, and other genes implicated in breast cancer. This chapter describes possible causes of breast cancer, why specific genes are implicated, a brief overview of how these genes were discovered, and the role mutations of specific genes are thought to play in the development of the disease. Chapter 5 considers issues of risk, prevention, screening, diagnosis, therapy (current and future), genetic testing, and genetic counseling. Chapter 6 describes current research with an emphasis on how the understanding of inherited breast cancer can be extrapolated to sporadic cases in the hope of designing better methods for prevention and therapy. The appendix lists resources for breast cancer patients and other interested readers.

Among the many sources I consulted during the writing of this book, the three major ones were *The Genetics of Cancer,* edited by B. J. Ponder and M. J. Waring (Kluwer Academic Publishers, 1995); *Breakthrough: The Race to Find the Breast Cancer Gene,* by K. Davies and M. White (John Wiley & Sons, Inc., 1996); and *Dr. Susan Love's Breast Book,* third edition, by Susan M. Love, M.D. with Karen Lindsey (Perseus Publishing, 2000).

Understanding Breast Cancer Genetics

1. Who Gets Breast Cancer?

The Rising Incidence of Breast Cancer

Breast cancer is a serious, potentially lethal disease. Its incidence has been rising steadily since 1950, most significantly in post-menopausal women. Approximately 183,000 new cases are diagnosed in the United States each year, comprising 31 percent of all cancers. Of these cases, over 40,000 will die. In fact, breast cancer is the leading cause of death in women forty to fifty-nine years old. An American woman today has a one in eight (12.5 percent) cumulative risk of developing breast cancer in her lifetime[1] (table 1.1).

Many theories have been proposed to explain the increased incidence of breast cancer in modern times. Some of the data may reflect the increase in life expectancy. The increase in reported cases may also reflect the increase in awareness and in screening programs for early cancers. However, these explanations do not fully account for the increased incidence. Researchers and clinicians agree only that breast cancer is a complex disease that reflects the interplay of environmental and genetic risk factors.

The Roles of Age, Sex, and Ethnicity

Although breast cancer can strike women in their twenties, it is primarily a disease of older age (table 1.2). At least 78 percent of patients are age fifty or older, and the incidence rate is increasing most rapidly in post-menopausal women. However, the incidence of breast cancer in women under age forty is also increasing. This is significant because the hormonal status of the female patient seems to play a role in the behavior of the disease. In younger women the tumors tend to be more aggressive, and the patients may have a less favorable prognosis.

Table 1.1 Cumulative risk of developing sporadic breast cancer by age		
Age	**Risk of Developing Breast Cancer**	**Percent Risk**
25	1 in 20,000	less than 0.5
30	1 in 2,500	less than 0.5
35	1 in 625	less than 0.5
40	1 in 215	less than 0.5
45	1 in 90	1.0
50	1 in 50	2.0
55	1 in 33	3.0
60	1 in 25	4.0
65	1 in 25	4.0
70	1 in 15	7.0
75	1 in 11	9.0
80	1 in 10	10.0
85	1 in 9	11.1
85+	1 in 8	12.5

Pregnant or lactating (nursing) women are not immune from breast cancer. It is, in fact, the most common cancer among this group of women, occurring in approximately one per 3000 pregnancies in women ages thirty-two to thirty-eight. The diagnosis of breast cancer during pregnancy is often complicated by the need to avoid certain types of chemotherapy and radiation, at least during the first trimester. These cancers are often not detected in the early, more curable stages.

Although the majority of breast cancer patients are women, in 1999 approximately 1,300 American men were diagnosed with the disease and approximately 400 died from it. Breast cancer follows a similar course in men and in women. However, since male breast

Table 1.2 Distribution of breast cancer cases by age	
Age	**Percent of Cases (based upon a representative sample)**
Under 50	22*
50–64	29
65–85+	49

* Only 6 percent of cases occur under age forty.

cancer is often diagnosed late, after the disease has progressed, men have a higher mortality rate. Treatment for male breast cancer is similar to treatment for women. Since breast cancer most commonly afflicts women, my focus in this book is on the female sex. However, principles discussed in this book are generally relevant to both sexes.

Some ethnic groups have a higher incidence of breast cancer than others. In the United States, the incidence is greater in non-Hispanic whites than in people of color. African-American women, however, are more likely to die of the disease, most likely because they may not receive an early diagnosis and treatment. Asian Americans who have lived in the United States for at least a decade have an 80 percent higher rate than those who recently immigrated. The incidence is also increasing among Native American women. The disease is nearly epidemic in many Western nations including the United States, Great Britain, Canada, and Israel. The incidence rate is also high in the Netherlands, Ireland, Denmark, and New Zealand. In contrast, the incidence rate is low in Mexico, Japan, Thailand, and China, as well as in some third-world countries in Africa and South America.

Role of Environment

Epidemiologists have noted that Japanese women, who normally have a low risk for developing breast cancer, eventually acquire the same risk as other Americans if they move to the United States. This observation and others suggest a role for environmental factors in the development of the disease. Scientists have studied the effects of exposure to many environmental and dietary factors that might contribute to the increasing incidence of breast cancer in Western countries. They have examined the effects of dietary fat, air and water pollutants, pesticides, radiation, alcohol, stress, oral contraceptives, hormone replacement therapy, and even abortions. They have also studied the effects of chemicals known as xenoestrogens, environmental chemicals that behave like estrogens. Organochlorines, for example, are common pollutants that exhibit estrogenic activity. These chemicals include PCBs, organic components of industrial waste that may leak into the water table. To date, none of the studies has revealed a specific environmental cause for breast cancer.

Risk Factors

While the link between environment and breast cancer remains unclear, a number of factors that increase the risk of developing the disease have been identified. The most important risk factor is age (table 1.1). A woman younger than fifty years, with no other risk factors, has only a 2 percent risk of developing the disease. In contrast, if she lives beyond eighty-five years, her risk is 12.5 percent. Other major risk factors include the age of menarche (first menstrual period), parity (number of pregnancies), whether she breast-fed her children, and age at menopause. These factors suggest a strong role for hormones, especially estrogens, in developing breast cancer. Use of hormone replacement therapy (HRT) over many years also increases risk, as may obesity and heavy ingestion of alcohol.

Women who inherit susceptibility to breast cancer (altered BRCA1 and BRCA2 genes, chapter 4) have a greater probability of developing the disease at a younger age. Their risk of contracting breast cancer by age fifty is 39 percent. Their lifetime risk of developing the disease is at least 56 percent. (Earlier estimates assessed the risk at 82 percent, but a careful review of the studies indicates that the risk may not be as great). Jewish women of Eastern European (Ashkenazi) ancestry have an increased risk of contracting inherited breast cancer compared to the general population.

Sporadic vs. Inherited Breast Cancer

In approximately 70 percent of cases, there is no family history of breast cancer. Those cancers are sporadic. The remaining 30 percent have a close family member (mother, sister, aunt) who also has the disease, suggesting that their susceptibility to developing the disease is inherited. However, a patient may have a close family member who is also affected and yet she may have sporadic disease. Only 5–10 percent of all breast cancer patients carry a known mutation that greatly enhances their chance of developing the disease. Sporadic breast cancers may also involve defective genes that enhance susceptibility, but to date these gene defects have not been clearly identified, nor are they known to be inherited. Although only some cancers are inherited, all involve damage to genes, as I will describe in chapter 2. Therefore, all cancers are genetic diseases.

Interplay of Genetics and Environment

Inheritance of susceptibility accounts for only a small percentage of breast cancers. In order for a cell to become cancerous, changes must occur in the genetic information that regulates its growth and relationship to nearby cells. These changes are most likely initiated by environmental events. However, even though most people in a geographic area are exposed to the same environmental insults, only a fraction will develop breast cancer. In the majority of the population, the triggering of cancer may be pure chance. An older person accumulates more environmental "insults" and eventually may sustain enough critical events to trigger the disease. However, if one has inherited a susceptibility to develop cancer, the same environmental insults may trigger the disease process sooner. Thus, although the greatest risks for developing breast cancer are being female, aging, and inheriting predisposing genes, environmental factors appear to be critically important in initiating the disease process.

2. What Is Breast Cancer?

An Introduction to Cancer Biology

In chapter 1, I introduced the concept of inherited versus sporadic breast cancer. In order to understand the role heredity plays in the development of the disease, it is important to understand what cancer is. Cancer is actually a catch-all term for many different diseases that share a fundamental defect: a loss of regulation of cell division and differentiation. This loss is generally due to the alteration of certain regulatory genes known as oncogenes and tumor suppressor genes. Cancer may therefore be considered a genetic disorder, even if the genetic alterations involved are not inherited.

Normal Cell Biology: Cell Division and Differentiation

Our bodies, and those of all living things except viruses (which are not always defined as living), are composed of basic units of structure and function known as cells. The two main compartments of cells are the nucleus and the cytoplasm. In most organisms, the genetic information is contained in molecules of deoxyribonucleic acid, or DNA (fig. 2.1). DNA is a long molecule consisting of a backbone of phosphates and sugars (deoxyribose) and various sequences of four possible nucleotide bases: adenine (A), thymine (T), guanine (G), and cytosine (C). Due to inherent chemical properties, A and T groups bind to each other, as do G and C groups. This property is called base pairing. DNA molecules exist as double strands wound in a helix formation. The phosphates and sugars provide the backbone, while base pairing binds the two strands to each other.

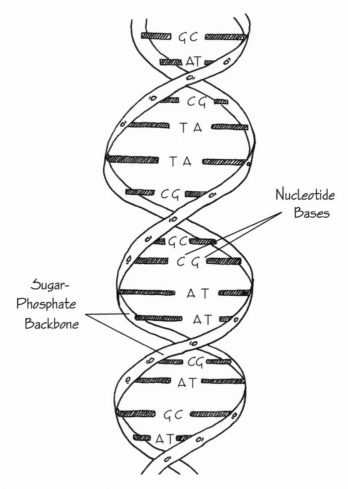

Fig. 2.1 The structure of DNA.

In the nucleus, the long strands of DNA are packaged into structures called chromosomes, which differ from each other by size and by patterns of staining when they are subjected to certain treatments. Chromosomes of a given species are displayed by pairs that express similar characteristics. Each pair is assigned a chromosome number. This type of display is called a karyotype.

Each chromosome consists of two strands known as chromatids, held together by a centromere. The centromere divides the chromosome into two arms, which are often unequal in length. The ends of chromosomes are also extremely important. These structures are called telomeres. When a cell divides, the telomeres shorten slightly. This phenomenon is linked to the finite lifespan of a given cell. When the telomeres become too short, the cell can no longer divide. Cancer cells, however, often produce an enzyme called telomerase that replaces the missing telomeres, thereby conferring immortality on the cell. Acquisition of immortality is one of the changes that occur in cells as they become cancerous.

Normal human cells have twenty-three pairs of similar (homologous) chromosomes, for a total of forty-six. One of each pair is derived from the individual's mother; the other, from the father. Chromosomes of each pair normally look alike, except for the X and Y chromosomes, which determine the sex of the individual.

Egg cells and sperm cells are unusual in that they only contain twenty-three chromosomes, or half the genetic information of other (somatic) cells. When an egg cell is fertilized by a sperm cell, the resulting fertilized cell, or zygote, contains a full complement of forty-six chromosomes and all the DNA of the new individual. The zygote soon divides, creating two daughter cells. Each daughter cell receives the same DNA as the parent cell. These two cells further divide into four, four into eight, and so forth, with each cell again receiving the same genetic information. The ability to reproduce genetic information faithfully is a major characteristic of cells. The growing cell mass begins to take on the shape we recognize as an embryo. Different cells begin to specialize—to become heart cells or lung cells or nerve cells. Although each cell has the full genetic information of the original fertilized egg, only some of the information is used by cells as they become specialized. This process is called differentiation. As cells become committed to a particular pathway of differentiation, they may continue to divide but have lost their omnipotence. For example, the progeny of a committed blood cell will never become a nerve cell.[2] Eventually, many cells become terminally differentiated and lose the ability to divide.

These cells senesce or die. New cells are created to take their place. Thus, cells serve specific functions in organisms, and most have finite lifespans.

Differentiated cells are organized into tissues such as muscle or nerves. Within a tissue, cells contact each other and communicate with each other through a variety of biochemical signals. Cells are often surrounded by a non-living extracellular matrix. Organs, such as heart or lung or stomach, are composed of combinations of tissues including a fibrous connective tissue scaffolding or stroma. The tissue cells enable the organs to perform their specific functions. The processes are tightly controlled by biochemical and nervous-system signals generated in various parts of the body.

Cells have specific growth characteristics depending upon the tissue and organ in which they are located. Some cells divide frequently, including those in hair follicles, precursor cells (stem cells) in bone marrow, and epithelial cells that line the gastrointestinal tract. Mature blood cells do not divide, but are replaced by the dividing precursor cells. Mature neurons (nerve cells) also do not divide, although recent evidence suggests that in adults there are immature neurons that can replenish worn-out cells. Other mature cells such as hepatocytes (liver cells) divide only when the organ is traumatized. If part of a liver is surgically removed for a transplant, the liver will soon grow back to its prior size. This growth is accomplished by rounds of synchronous cell division, in which all cells divide at the same time.

Before a cell divides, it replicates its genetic information, or DNA. The cell goes through a process known as the cell cycle that has its own defined stages. The non-dividing or resting cell is in a state known as G_0 (G for gap) in which the cell carries out its normal metabolic functions. When cultures of quiescent, non-dividing cells are fixed (preserved) and stained with dyes that distinguish the nuclei from the cytoplasm, the nuclei may have a coarse, granular appearance under a microscope but the chromosomes are not distinct. In response to specific signals, the cell enters a state called G_1 in which it makes the molecules involved in the replication of DNA and other cellular components. The cell then enters S (for synthesis) phase in which the DNA is replicated. At this point, the cell contains twice the amount of DNA as a resting cell. The chromosomes are still not distinct. When all necessary molecules have been synthesized, and after another pause, G_2, the cell enters the M (mitosis) phase (fig. 2.2).

The process of mitosis consists of five stages. The first is called interphase, during which time the events of the cell cycle from G_0 through G_2 occur. The nucleus is surrounded by a distinct nuclear membrane. The chromosomes are not distinct, but there is a prominent round structure in the nucleus called the nucleolus. Two other prominent structures, the centrioles, may be seen in the cytoplasm. In the second stage, prophase, the chromosomes condense and each appears as two identical chromatids held together by a centromere. Each chromatid contains a double-stranded molecule of DNA. The nuclear membrane and nucleolus disappear. The centrioles move to opposite poles of the cell, and ray-like structures called mitotic spindles form between them. Other rays called asters surround each centriole. The chromosomes migrate to the equator of the cell. In the third stage, metaphase, the centromere of each double-stranded chromosome attaches to the mitotic spindle at the equator of the cell. In the fourth stage, anaphase, the centromeres divide. Each half-centromere and its attached chromatid moves along the spindle toward the nearest centriole so that one chromatid of each pair ends up at each pole. In the fifth stage, telophase, the cell physically divides at the equator, the mitotic spindle and aster rays disappear, the centrioles divide, the chromosomes become less distinct, and the nuclear membrane and nucleolus reappear. Thus, a single cell has given rise to two daughter cells containing the identical genetic information that was in the original parent cell. The cells enter interphase and the cell cycle begins again.

Cell division is an exquisitely controlled process. Progression through the cell cycle is regulated by checkpoints at the boundary between G_1 and S and during G_2. Under normal conditions, a cell will not enter S phase until it has made all the molecules necessary for DNA synthesis. Likewise, if an error occurs in this synthesis, the cell will not progress through G_2 to M until the error is repaired. Special proteins known as proofreading and repair enzymes check

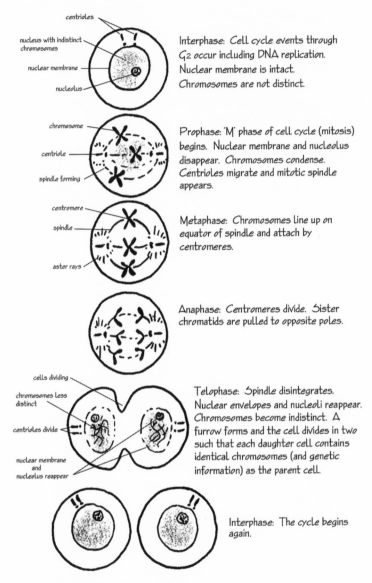

centrioles

nucleus with indistinct chromosomes

nuclear membrane

nucleolus

Interphase: Cell cycle events through G2 occur including DNA replication. Nuclear membrane is intact. Chromosomes are not distinct.

chromosome

centriole

spindle forming

Prophase: 'M' phase of cell cycle (mitosis) begins. Nuclear membrane and nucleolus disappear. Chromosomes condense. Centrioles migrate and mitotic spindle appears.

centromere

spindle

aster rays

Metaphase: Chromosomes line up on equator of spindle and attach by centromeres.

Anaphase: Centromeres divide. Sister chromatids are pulled to opposite poles.

cells dividing

chromosomes less distinct

centrioles divide

nuclear membrane and nucleolus reappear

Telophase: Spindle disintegrates. Nuclear envelopes and nucleoli reappear. Chromosomes become indistinct. A furrow forms and the cell divides in two such that each daughter cell contains identical chromosomes (and genetic information) as the parent cell.

Interphase: The cycle begins again.

Fig. 2.2 Schematic depiction of the stages of mitosis.

for accuracy at checkpoints along the cell cycle pathway, and may correct the error. Alternatively, the cell may activate a genetically programmed sequence of events that cause the cell to die. This "suicide" program is known as apoptosis. The systems of checkpoints, proofreading, repair, and apoptosis ensure that daughter cells receive correct genetic information from the parent cells and that, if they don't, they die.

Derangements of the Cell Cycle and the Rise of Malignant Cells

Cancers often arise when errors (mutations) occur in replicating DNA. Some of these errors are fatal to the cell and trigger apoptosis. Often, however, the mutations are not lethal. In time, cells may acquire multiple errors, and the controls regulating the progression through the cell cycle fail. If a cell begins to divide inappropriately, so that its progeny cells accumulate more quickly than surrounding cells, a mass of cells may form within the tissue. This is the beginning of a tumor. The cells themselves may still be relatively normal, and the tumor is benign. It may occupy space but it does not invade normal tissue. The cells may still carry out their normal differentiated functions. There is also evidence of cross-talk between the altered cells and the normal stroma (connective tissue framework) in which they are found. The stroma sends chemical signals to the cells and may keep their errant behavior in check. However, the cells may eventually begin to exhibit changes in behavior so that they do not function as normal cells in the tissue and organ in which they are located. The altered cells may no longer distribute their genetic information evenly between daughter cells as they divide, and they become increasingly genetically unstable. Eventually, cells acquire the ability to invade normal tissue. Cells exhibiting numerous, progressive genetic alterations and invasive potential are malignant. These cells have crossed a threshold beyond which they no longer respond to normal regulatory signals and controls. Cancers are growths or tumors composed of malignant cells, and have the potential to invade normal tissue.

Cancers are usually clonal in origin; that is, they arise from a single cell. Each altered daughter cell may acquire other mutations, and pass these changes to its own progeny. In time, the mass of cancerous cells will show considerable variability. This phenomenon is called tumor heterogeneity, and may influence the course of the disease.

A principle of evolution, "survival of the fittest," applies to the developing malignant tumor. In evolution, an organism that has acquired traits that increase its ability to survive in a given environment is said to have a "selective advantage." In cancer biology, tumor cells that acquire mutations for rapid, independent growth, invasion of normal tissue, and the ability to spread to distant sites have a great selective advantage. In a heterogeneous tumor, there is a strong probability that at least one tumor cell will acquire the mutations that enable the tumor to spread.

Malignant cells that spread have acquired the ability to break free of their surroundings and invade blood and lymphatic vessels. This activity requires that the cells activate genes for enzymes that can break down the extracellular matrix that holds the cells in place in a tissue. Alternatively, changes may occur in the surrounding stroma to allow the altered cells to escape. This latter theory is currently the subject of experimental inquiry. If the cancer cells can successfully escape into the circulation and survive there, they may then travel to distant sites and invade other tissues and organs. This process of invasion and acquiring the ability to survive in a "foreign" environment is known as metastasis. Certain cancers have a pattern for metastasizing to specific sites that cannot be explained simply by the distribution of blood vessels and lymphatics that drain the tumors. For example, breast cancer often metastasizes to underarm lymph nodes and then to brain, lung, ovaries, and bone. Current studies suggest that tumor cells express specific proteins on their surface that recognize specific protein sequences on the cells lining the lymphatic and blood vessels. Binding of the tumor cells to these vessel cells causes changes in the vessels that permit the tumor cells to escape the circulation at that site. The process by which a tumor develops from a single damaged cell to metastatic cancer is called tumor progression.

A malignant tumor requires an adequate blood supply to support the metabolic demands of its growing mass. The tumor cells secrete substances called angiogenesis factors (e.g., vascular endothelial growth factor, or veg-f), which recruit new blood vessels into the tumor. Metastatic tumors must also develop an adequate blood supply in their new site.

Metastatic cancer cells no longer perform any differentiated function in the tissues and organs they invade. They grow at the expense of that tissue, and ultimately destroy it. It is often the destruction of vital organs by metastatic cancer cells that leads to the death of the afflicted person.

Since the body consists of many different types of cells, many different types of cancers can arise. Some cancers are more aggressive than others. Some are more common in children; others, in adults. However, all arise in cells that are undergoing division. The primary defect must be passed on to other cells in order for the tumor to become established.

The Anatomy of the Human Breast: Where Breast Cancers Begin

In order to understand the nature of different cancers, it is helpful to understand the structures of the organs and tissues in which they arise. As seen in fig. 2.3, the human breast tissue consists of special glands called lobules that surround branches of ducts like leaves on a tree. Each breast contains six to nine independent ductal systems that run from the nipple back to the underlying pectoral muscle. The amount of breast tissue is genetically determined, and may extend from the collarbone to the lowest ribs and from the breastbone to the back of the armpit. Milk is made in the lobules and is then transported through the ducts to the nipple. Breast cancers most often begin in the cells that line the ducts. These lining

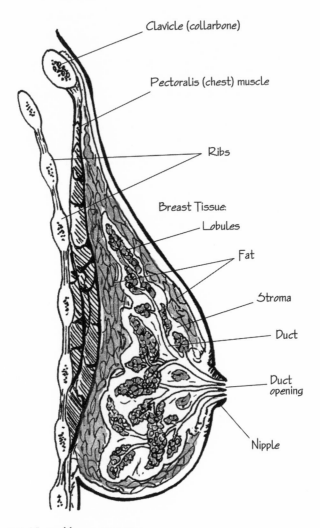

Fig. 2.3 Normal breast anatomy.

cells, like all lining and surface cells, are called epithelial cells. Cancers of epithelial cells are called carcinomas.

The lobules and ducts are embedded in a stroma of fat and fibrous connective tissue, nerves, blood vessels, and lymphatic

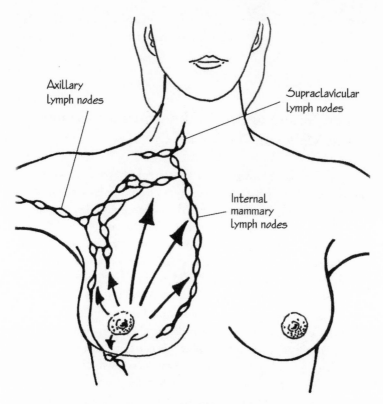

Fig. 2.4 Lymphatic system draining the human female breast.

vessels. The lymphatic vessels drain fluid containing waste materials from the breast into a series of filters called lymph nodes (fig. 2.4). These are situated under the armpit (axillary lymph nodes), under the breastbone (internal mammary lymph nodes), and above the collarbone (supraclavicular lymph nodes). The nodes contain collections of immune system cells that detect and destroy invading foreign organisms and antigens (substances that elicit an immune response). When breast cancers spread, the cells tend to invade the lymphatics and travel to the axillary nodes. Surgeons will often removed a number of nodes to check for the presence of malignant cells. The presence or absence of cancer cells in these nodes is important for determining treatment options and prognosis.

The Nature of Breast Abnormalities: Benign and Malignant Lesions

Breast lumps and irregularities are extremely common. Many women have lumpy breasts and are often told they have a condition known as fibrocystic change in which benign, fluid-filled cysts or excessive growth of fibrous, connective tissue occur.[3] These lumps tend to grow and shrink with the menstrual cycle, and may be associated with cyclical breast tenderness and even nipple discharge. Younger women often develop a solid but benign tumor known as a fibroadenoma, which consists of glandular and fibrous tissue. These, too, are benign. However, some abnormal breast conditions and lumps have a higher probability of progressing to malignancy. A condition called "atypical hyperplasia" is correlated with increased cancer risk. In this condition, there is an overgrowth of the ductal epithelium, and the cells are not quite normal in microscopic appearance. It is therefore important that a physician check out palpable, persistent lumps. In pre-menopausal women, approximately 8 percent of breast lumps are malignant, in contrast to 50 percent of the lumps in post-menopausal women. True cancers are often accompanied by a scarlike fibrous reaction to the growing lump and feel hard to the touch. They do not come and go during the menstrual cycle.

Breast cancers vary in biological behavior (for example, their growth rate) and tendency to metastasize. The least dangerous are those that arise in the lobule itself and do not spread. They are often found in both breasts (bilateral), but may never cause the patient any problems other than worry. This form of breast cancer is known as LCIS, or lobular carcinoma in situ. Some question whether they are true malignancies or markers of a potential malignancy that may or may not occur. LCIS itself cannot usually be detected by mammogram or even by physical examination, and is often an incidental finding during surgery for other breast conditions. LCIS is associated with a 25 percent risk of invasive cancer over twenty-five years, at which time they become detectable on mammograms. LCIS patients must therefore be monitored regularly to detect invasive cancer at the earliest possible time.

Tumors that arise in the epithelium of the ducts can remain within the duct and are known as DCIS, or ductal carcinoma in situ. DCIS can acquire the ability to invade beyond the duct into the stroma. The most common breast cancer (80 percent of all breast cancers) is invasive ductal carcinoma. It may grow and invade locally, or it may travel through the lymphatics to other parts of the body. It is the danger of metastasis that makes this form of cancer such a concern. Other, less common breast cancers include medullary, colloid, tubular, and adenoid cystic carcinomas. These generally have a good prognosis. In contrast, another rare breast cancer, "inflammatory" carcinoma, is usually deadly within two years of diagnosis. Inflammatory carcinoma spreads through the lymphatics of the skin and disseminates widely and rapidly. Paget's disease of the nipple (nipple cancer) also has a poor prognosis.

Biology of Sporadic vs. Hereditary Breast Cancer

Recent studies have demonstrated that hereditary breast cancers often present different histological characteristics from those that occur sporadically. However, the biological behavior of tumors is often the same. In fact, younger women with hereditary breast cancer often do better than those whose tumors arise sporadically. Women who have two or more first degree relatives (mother, sister) with breast cancer have a greatly increased chance of developing the disease at a younger age, but the disease itself is not necessarily more aggressive. Overall mortality rates are similar between patients with hereditary breast cancer and those whose tumors arise spontaneously.

The Role of Sex, Age, Hormonal Status, and Ethnicity on the Biology of Breast Cancer

As noted in chapter 1, men are also susceptible to breast cancer, and it can be just as deadly. The disease follows a similar course, but since men are often unaware that they can get breast cancer they may delay seeing a doctor when they find a suspicious lump, and therefore may be diagnosed too late for effective treatment.

Age is the greatest risk factor for developing breast cancer, but tumors in post-menopausal women are sometimes less aggressive than in those who are pre-menopausal.

A role for female sex hormones in breast cancer has long been suspected because women are far more susceptible than men. Early menarche and late menopause, which lengthen the period of exposure to sex hormones, increase the risk for breast cancer. The age at which a woman has her first child, the number of pregnancies, and whether she breast feeds may also be risk factors and are related to hormonal status. The amount of breast tissue available may be a factor, but small-breasted women are at similar risk to those with large breasts.

Many breast cancers are sensitive to female sex hormones such as estrogen and progesterone. Estrogen and possibly progesterone may stimulate breast cancers that have already begun to grow (promoter effects) rather than cause the disease. It used to be thought that estrogen and progesterone bind to specific receptors on the surface of the malignant cells, then enter the cells and provide biochemical signals that stimulate them to proliferate. In recent years, researchers have discovered that there are two types of estrogen receptors. The "classical" estrogen receptor is now designated alpha, and another receptor, discovered in 1995, is designated beta. Some tissues express both alpha and beta receptors. The beta receptor exists in all tissues that express alpha receptors but also in some tissues that do not. Estrogens can act on alpha and beta receptors independently or in combination, and can have either stimulatory or inhibitory effects on the cells depending upon the specific receptor that is bound. In other words, estrogen may stimulate cells to proliferate or may prevent the proliferation. The effect of estrogen depends upon the form of the hormone and the receptor it binds to.

Drugs that bind the alpha or beta receptors can act as estrogen agonists (mimics) in some tissues and antagonists in others. The different properties of these receptors are the basis for a class of drugs called selective estrogen receptor modulators (SERMs). The drugs tamoxifen and raloxifene are compounds of that class, and are antagonists of estrogen in breast tissue. They are sometimes called anti-estrogens.

The effect of progesterone is also mediated by different receptors (PR-A and PR-B) and is influenced by the presence or absence of estrogen. Progesterone by itself inhibits the growth of breast cancer cells studied in the laboratory by inducing cell cycle arrest in G_1. In the presence of estrogens, however, progesterone can stimulate growth by increasing sensitivity to estrogen or to other growth factors. Estrogen receptors increase the expression of progesterone receptors. In vivo, progesterone stimulates both the maturation and proliferation of breast epithelium and is known to regulate expression of many other growth-related genes. The effects of progesterone on breast epithelium are obviously complex. Its role in breast cancer is still being investigated.

Although some ethnic groups have higher rates of breast cancer than others, the biology of the disease is not necessarily different between the groups. The type of cells involved, the size and location at diagnosis, and the course of treatment are more likely to influence the course of disease and the eventual outcome. African-American women have a lower incidence of breast cancer than American white women, but have a higher rate of fatalities from the disease. This is likely due to socioeconomic factors leading to a delay in diagnosis until the disease has already spread.

How Does Breast Cancer Spread?

As indicated above, breast cancers usually begin in the epithelium lining the ducts and break through the walls of these structures into the surrounding stroma. Since numerous blood and lymphatic vessels penetrate the stroma, cancer cells that invade these vessels can travel throughout the body and then invade other organs. By the time a tumor is 0.3–0.5 cm. (0.1–0.2 inches) in size and detectable by mammogram, it may have been growing for nine years! A palpable tumor is usually 1.0–1.5 cm. (0.4–0.6 inches) in size and contains 100 million cells.

How Does Breast Cancer Kill?

Once a cancer has spread, it is difficult to control. Treatments such as surgery, chemotherapy, or radiation may reduce the mass of the tumor, but metastatic cells may remain in lymph nodes or elsewhere and eventually resume their rampage. Some cells develop resistance to chemotherapy or radiation. Those cells have a selective advantage and will continue to grow. Eventually, vital organs are destroyed and the patient dies of organ failure or hemorrhage. Cancer patients often develop fatal infections. White blood cells, which are critical for fighting infections, are made in the bone marrow. As mentioned above, chemotherapy destroys all fast-dividing cells including those in the marrow. The patients are left immunosuppressed and are susceptible to a variety of infections that people with intact immune systems normally overcome. The marrow may also be destroyed by direct invasion by the tumor cells. It is therefore extremely important for breast cancer—or any fast-growing cancer—to be detected early, before the cells have invaded the circulatory and lymphatic systems.

Survival Paradox

Some patients succumb quickly to breast cancer despite aggressive treatment, while others live in apparent good health for many years. In addition, some patients do well for a number of years after treatment and then suffer a recurrence of their cancers. There are no easy explanations for these observations. I discussed earlier that tumor cells make angiogenesis factors (substances that induce blood vessel growth) that sustain the tumor. Primary tumors also secrete angiostatins, which antagonize formation of such blood vessels. If a primary tumor is surgically removed after it has metastasized, the source of angiostatins is also removed, and metastatic cells are no longer inhibited from secreting angiogenesis factors that promote blood vessel formation and the establishment of new tumors. Alternatively, the metastatic cells may stay dormant in their new site until some new mutation or other stimulus triggers them to grow.

Each individual is unique and so is his or her disease. Some tumors are more aggressive than others. In younger, pre-menopausal women, tumors not displaying receptors for estrogen and/or proges-terone often tend to be more aggressive and metastasize more rap-idly. Some tumors do not appear to be aggressive, but metastasize early. It used to be thought that if a woman was cancer-free for five years after treatment, she had beaten the disease. Today we know of recurrences after a decade. Again, the importance of early detection and aggressive treatment must be stressed. In chapter 5, I offer some insight into current detection and treatment methods.

3. The Roles of Genes Versus Inheritance

What is a Gene? What is its Role in a Cell?

In previous chapters, I discussed the importance of faithful replication of DNA to the normal activity of cells in tissues and organs. I suggested that cancer may occur if this process is impaired. In this chapter, I explain in greater detail why abnormal replication of DNA and the genetic information it contains can be so detrimental.

As you know, genetic information is encoded in genes, which are composed of DNA. A gene consists of a specific sequence of DNA bases; that is, a particular linear arrangement of As, Ts, Cs, and Gs that codes for a specific protein. The location of a gene is designated by which of the twenty-three chromosome pairs it is on, whether it is on the short or long arm of the chromosome, and how close it is to the centromere. That site is called a locus. Since there are two copies of every gene, each copy is located at the same locus on one of the homologous chromosomes that form the pair.

Genes are essentially blueprints for proteins. Proteins consist of building blocks called amino acids. Animal (including human) proteins contain combinations of twenty different amino acids. The coding region of a gene determines the linear sequence of amino acids that form the protein. The code is "read" in groups of three DNA bases such as GTT and determines which amino acid (GTT codes for valine) is next in line to join the growing chain. The DNA base triplet that codes for an amino acid is called a codon.

Some proteins determine the structure of cells. Other proteins, or enzymes, control most of the cell's metabolic activities. Proteins also form part of the extracellular scaffolding that holds cells and tissues together. Proteins such as albumin circulate in the blood-stream and carry other biologically important molecules from one site to another. Proper function of genes and their protein products are necessary for life. If a mutation occurs in the blueprint (the gene), the protein it codes for may be defective and may not be able to do its job. The protein may not be produced at all. Sometimes too much protein is produced or may be produced at the wrong time. Mutations can therefore lead to disease and even to death because of their effects on proteins.

The total genetic information in a species is called the genome. The Human Genome Project is a government-supported program whose mission is to identify and map the location of all the genes in the human genome. Once the genes are identified, the proteins they code for can be discerned. Manipulation of these genes and proteins will provide a better understanding of disease processes and may enable the development of new prevention strategies and cures. A brand new field called proteomics is already applying genomic knowledge to how proteins function in normal and in disease states.

Although human cells contain approximately three billion base pairs of DNA, the results of the Human Genome Project suggest that there are only approximately 35,000 genes. DNA can be visualized as a linear arrangement of As, Ts, Cs, and Gs. The order of nucleotide bases in the sequence is absolutely critical. A change in any base is called a mutation and could lead to major consequences for the cell, and possibly for the individual. Although the DNA is arranged in this linear sequence of bases, most of the DNA does not serve as a template for the protein the gene produces. A linear stretch of DNA may serve as a coding region, but may be followed by another stretch that does not seem to code for anything, and whose role is not yet understood. Another coding region may follow. Non-coding regions within a gene are called introns; coding regions are called exons. Mutations in exons are usually more critical than those in introns or other non-coding regions. Some sequences of DNA are important for regulation of gene expression (see the following paragraph). Others indicate where a gene—and therefore its protein product—begins and where it ends.

Although all cells in an individual contain the same genes, not all genes function in all cells or at the same time. Gene activity, or expression, is a highly regulated process. Some genes code for proteins that are necessary for the normal metabolic functions of a cell. These genes are always active (constitutively expressed). In contrast, other genes are active only at specific times such as during cell division or after dinner. Their expression is regulated by the binding of small regulatory protein molecules to specific DNA sequences known as promoters and enhancers that lie near each gene. Some regulatory proteins turn the genes on; others turn them off. In many situations, the on-off switch is reversible. However, in the process of cellular differentiation, the biochemical events that turned a gene off were once thought to be irreversible, and the cell was thought to be committed to a specific differentiation pathway. We now know from cloning experiments on adult animals that, given the proper environment, these genes can be turned on again.[4]

An analogy to gene expression may be seen in the operation of a computer. The computer has a hard drive and an operating system, and contains programs and files in its memory. The programs are always there, but they are not always operating. They are stored in discontinuous sites on the hard drive. The person using the computer selects the specific program and opens the program files when they are needed. The computer uses internal operations to open these files as continuous units. These files can then be stored again in the computer's memory. However, these files sometimes become damaged or corrupted and cannot be retrieved. Sometimes the errors can be corrected, but at other times they can cause the whole hard drive to crash.

In this analogy, the cell is the hard drive. Constitutive genes behave like the operating system and are necessary for the cell to function. DNA is the memory. All of the programs (non-constitutive genes) are there, although not necessarily in continuous order and not always operating. When a cell needs to open a program (express a gene), it goes through a series of internal operations to produce the executable program files (proteins) and their necessary sub-files (amino acids). If any of these steps is corrupted, the program will not operate properly, and may affect the entire cell (hard drive). The damage may or may not be repairable, and the cell may ultimately die (hard drive crash).

The "internal operations" that a cell uses to read the genetic code, and ultimately to synthesize a specific protein, are called transcription and translation (fig. 3.1). In transcription, the sequence of DNA that constitutes a gene is transcribed into RNA. RNA is structurally similar to DNA, but contains uracil (U) instead of thymine (T), and the sugar is ribose rather than deoxyribose. This RNA is a single-stranded rather than double-stranded molecule. The RNA is then processed into messenger RNA (mRNA). Processing includes the excision of introns and the addition of structures known as a cap and a tail. The mRNA is then exported to the cytoplasm, where it lines up on structures known as ribosomes to be translated into protein.

Translation involves a small molecule known as transfer RNA (tRNA). tRNA contains three linearly arranged bases at one end known as an anti-codon. The anti-codon binds three linearly arranged RNA bases, or a triplet codon, on mRNA by complementary base pairing. In other words, if a DNA codon sequence was GTT, the corresponding mRNA sequence is CAA and the anti-codon on the tRNA is GUU. The tRNA carries a specific amino acid at its other end. The anti-codon determines which of twenty possible amino acids a particular tRNA molecule carries. The amino acids combine to form a small polypeptide chain. Multiple polypeptide chains combine to form functioning proteins. The linear arrangement of bases in DNA therefore determines the sequence of mRNA. The mRNA sequence determines the binding of tRNA molecules carrying specific amino acids. If a mutation occurs in the DNA, the error will be copied into the mRNA and the wrong amino acid may be added to the growing polypeptide chain. The linear arrangement of amino acids determines the structure of a protein and is crucial to the ultimate function of the protein in a cell. As mentioned above, the protein may be structural, or may be an enzyme that catalyzes a biochemical reaction. If either the structural protein or the enzyme is not properly made, the results could be disastrous.

Cells do not exist in a vacuum. They receive signals from adjacent and distant cells through a highly integrated network.

Transcription

I. DNA is transcribed to RNA in nucleus.
2. RNA is processed into mRNA and exported to cytoplasm.

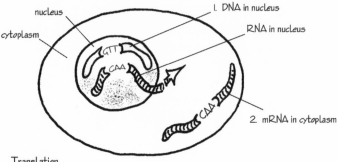

Translation

3. tRNA carries amino acid to mRNA.
4. Ribosome moves along mRNA.
5. tRNA binds to mRNA, deposits amino acid to growing polypeptide chain, and moves off to pick another amino acid.

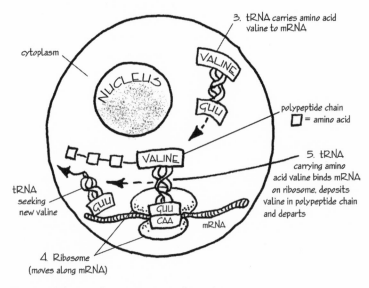

Fig. 3.1 Scheme of transcription and translation.

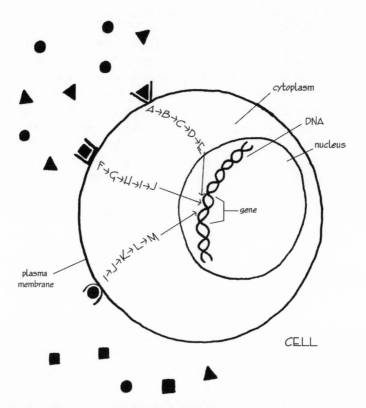

Fig. 3.2 Schematic depicition of a signal transduction cascade. The cell receives multiple signals from various regulatory factors (circles, triangles, squares). Each factor binds to a specific type of surface receptor. Each type of receptor is linked to a series of specific molecular events (A→B→C etc.) that convey the signal to the cell's nucleus. Depending upon the specific signal pathway, small regulatory proteins bind to the region of DNA that controls the transcription of a specific gene. Integration of multiple complex signals leads to changs in gene expression.

This network depends upon specific cell surface proteins (receptors) that bind biochemical messengers. When a messenger molecule binds its receptor, a cascade of molecular signals is sent to the nucleus to modify gene expression. This process is called signal transduction (fig. 3.2). A given cell may have many receptors on its surface, each linked to different signal transduction pathways. These signals must be integrated for the ultimate fate of the cell to be determined. If a cell has genetic damage, the response of the cell to a given set of signals may be inappropriate. If the damaged cell survives, its progeny also faces possibly faulty integration of multiple signals, which is then repeated in subsequent rounds of cell division. The combination of genetic damage and faulty response to controlling cell signals may lead to the development of cancer.

Not all mutations are harmful. Normal variability in the genome allows for the variability of individuals. Although the genes on homologous chromosomes are similar, they may not be identical. This variability results usually from inherited mutations in genes that are not harmful or may even be advantageous. Evolution depends upon them. Normal variation means that at a given locus, a gene may be one of multiple forms or alleles. The collection of specific alleles in an individual is known as the genotype. The collection of gene products is known as the phenotype.

Some alleles are dominant, so that they determine phenotype. Other alleles are recessive, and the effect of their protein products is seen only if both alleles at that locus are recessive. For example, let us assume in humans that brown eyes are dominant and blue eyes are recessive[5] (fig. 3.3). An individual receives one gene from his father and one from his mother. A brown-eyed parent may have two dominant alleles for brown eyes (BB) or one dominant and one recessive (Bb). A blue-eyed parent will only have recessive alleles (bb). If the child inherits B alleles from both parents, or a B from one and b from the other, it will have brown eyes (BB or Bb). If it inherits the b allele from each parent, it will have blue eyes (bb). Some alleles, however, are expressed in co-dominant fashion, each contributing to the overall phenotype. For example, let us assume that hazel eyes reflect a combination of brown and blue alleles, where brown is not totally dominant so that blue also exerts some effect. (In reality, this may not be the case.) The overall effect of a gene on the phenotype is referred to as the penetrance of the gene. By definition, genes that are inherited in dominant

Fig. 3.3 The effects of dominant, recessive, and co-dominant genes on eye color. We will assume that brown is dominant and blue is recessive. Homozygous (BB) and heterozygous (Bb) individuals have brown eyes. Only homozygous (bb) individuals have blue eyes. However, if genes for brown eyes and blue eyes were co-dominant, the eye color of a individual would be between brown and blue depending upon the relative penetrance of each gene.

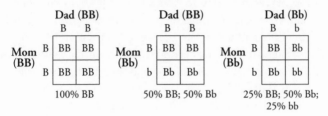

a. Both parents have brown eyes. Brown eyes can be BB or Bb. If both parents are BB, all children will be brown-eyed and BB. If one parent is BB and the other, Bb, all children will have brown eyes. However, each child has a 50 percent chance of being BB and 50 percent of being heterozygous Bb. If both parents are Bb, each child has a 25 percent chance of being brown-eyed and BB, a 50 percent chance of being brown-eyed and Bb, and a 25 percent chance of being blue-eyed (bb).

	Dad (BB)				**Dad (Bb)**	
	B	B			B	b
Mom b	Bb	Bb		**Mom** b	Bb	bb
(bb) b	Bb	Bb		**(bb)** b	Bb	bb
	100% Bb				50% Bb; 50% bb	

b. One parent has brown eyes; the other has blue eyes. Brown eyes can be BB or Bb; blue eyes are bb and recessive. If brown-eyed parent is BB, all children will be Bb and will have brown eyes. If the brown-eyed parent is Bb, each child will have a 50 percent chance of being blue-eyed (bb) or brown-eyed (Bb).

	Dad (bb)	
	b	b
Mom b	bb	bb
(bb) b	bb	bb
	100% bb	

c. Both parents have blue eyes. Blue eyes are bb (recessive). All children have blue eyes (bb).

(or recessive) autosomal fashion are not located on the X chromosome. Genes located on the X chromosome are always dominant in males since the Y chromosome does not contain homologous alleles.

Although DNA is usually copied faithfully, there are opportunities for genetic information to "mix and match." This process is important for evolution and allows for the diversity of individuals within a species and ultimately, the specific traits that define a species. Genetic scrambling occurs frequently during meiosis, which is the process by which gametes (egg and sperm cells) are made. Gametes are derived from special cells known as germ cells. In meiosis, several events occur. Following an initial round of division that is similar to what occurs in mitosis, the cells undergo a special type of cell division known as a reduction division. During this process, the homologous chromosomes line up but do not duplicate. Instead, they separate into daughter cells, so that each carries only twenty-three chromosomes and, therefore, a single copy of each gene. During meiosis, exchanges of DNA occur between homologous chromosomes prior to reduction division. This process is known as recombination. The further apart two genes are located on a given chromosome, the more likely a recombination event will occur between them. As a result, each gamete will contain some genes from the individual's mother and some from its father.

Non-gamete (somatic) cells containing a full complement of DNA are diploid, whereas gametes, containing only half of the DNA, are haploid. When the haploid egg cell is fertilized by the haploid sperm cell, the resulting zygote is diploid, containing a full complement of DNA, forty-six chromosomes, and two alleles of each gene. One allele is derived from the egg, the other from the sperm. However, the egg and sperm cells will contain a random combination of specific alleles derived from the female and male that produced them. The resulting combination will result in a zygote with its unique combination of alleles and therefore a unique phenotype. That is why, except for single-egg twins (and other clones), no two individuals are identical.

Damage to Genes: Germline vs. Somatic Mutations; Error Corrections, Consequences

In addition to the natural "genetic scrambling" that takes place during DNA replication, errors can also occur (see chapter 2). Approximately one error occurs per million base pairs of DNA being replicated. Since there are approximately three billion base pairs in the human genome, each time a cell replicates it may have as many as 3,000 errors. Obviously, this is a dangerously high rate of error, and cells have evolved highly accurate proofreading and repair systems to deal with it.

As mentioned in chapter 2, errors in DNA replication are called mutations. The many types of mutations include substitution of one base for another, deletion of bases, repetition of bases, and inversion of bases. Frame shift mutations occur when insertions and deletions of bases (other than multiples of three) alter all codons that follow, leading to a non-functional protein. Some genetic errors occur at the level of the chromosome. Some chromosomal mutations involve translocations, where a section of a chromosome is moved to another position on the same chromosome or to another chromosome. Others involve non-disjunction, where a pair of chromosomes fails to separate during meiosis. The resulting gamete therefore contains an extra chromosome. Upon fertilization, the resulting zygote has three copies of a chromosome rather than two. Trisomy 21 (in which there are three copies of chromosome 21) causes Down syndrome, a common cause of mental retardation. At the time of meiosis, the two chromosomes 21 fail to dissociate, so the resulting egg or sperm cell has two copies instead of one. When the defective gamete combines with a normal egg or sperm, the resultant zygote receives another copy of the chromosome and of all the genes located on it. The effect of expression of all of these genes causes the phenotypic changes associated with the syndrome. At least 2,000 diseases have been associated with mutations in single genes, and perhaps an equal number are linked to other mutations. Approximately 100 genes have been associated with cancer. Chromosomal anomalies, especially translocations, are also often associated with cancer.

Damage to genes may result from exposure to mutagens such as pesticides, tobacco smoke, and radiation, or they may occur randomly during DNA synthesis and cell division. As described in chapter 2, cells have built-in damage-control and repair systems, so the damage is usually repaired or the cell is destroyed by apoptosis. The damage control system, unfortunately, is not 100 percent foolproof. The genes coding for the repair enzymes may themselves be mutated. Mutations can also occur at the level of the small proteins that regulate transcription and translation, or those that transduce signals from the cell surface to the genes in the nucleus. It is important to remember that mutations occur both in somatic cells and germ cells, and that some result in cancer.

Although mutations can occur in any cell that divides, only germline mutations can be passed on to future generations. Somatic mutations, however, can give rise to diseases within the individual. For example, a non-lethal mutation may occur in an egg or sperm cell. The resulting offspring of that gamete will carry the mutation in every somatic and germ cell. Whether or not the effect of the mutated gene is seen will depend upon its penetrance (the effect of a gene on the phenotype) and the effect of the homologous allele contributed by the other parent. A somatic mutation, in contrast, may be expressed and harmful to an individual, but will not be passed to future generations.

Special Genes Involved in Cancer: Oncogenes and Tumor Suppressor Genes

Mutations involved in initiation of cancer often occur in genes regulating the cell cycle. Two major regulatory classes of genes have been discovered. One group is known as oncogenes, due to their potential to cause cancer. In normal cells, these genes are called proto-oncogenes and are normal genes that make the cells go into the cell cycle and divide. Many code for proteins that are growth factors for cells or receptors for such factors. Examples are the receptors for epidermal growth factor (EGF) or its truncated (shortened) version, Her2/neu. Mutations in proto-oncogenes may cause uncontrolled growth of cells by cell division, leading to cancer.

Certain viruses contain oncogenes and are capable of causing cancer in animals, and more rarely in humans. Mutated oncogenes in humans were first thought to be viral in origin. We now know that the viruses pick up normal cellular proto-oncogenes and incorporate the DNA sequences into their own genomes, where they acquire the ability to disrupt the cell cycle and cause cancer.

Tumor suppressor genes are cell cycle regulators that make the cell stop dividing, and may induce apoptosis. Mutations in these genes may inhibit their function, thereby causing the cell to divide uncontrollably. Normally, cell division is exquisitely balanced by growth and suppressor stimuli. Derangement of either "go" or "stop" signals can lead to inappropriate cell division and cancer.

Several tumor suppressor genes are associated with specific cancers including breast cancer. These include BRCA1, BRCA2 (breast cancer genes 1 and 2), and p53 (a protein product of a tumor suppressor gene). I will discuss these in greater detail in the following chapter. For now, it is sufficient to understand that these genes are part of the normal human genome and play a role in regulating cell division. If these genes are disrupted and do not function properly, the consequences may include the development of cancer.

Some genes expressed by cancer cells prevent the induction of apoptosis, which would normally destroy a genetically damaged cell. An example of such a gene is BCL2. Some types of chemotherapy damage a cell's DNA and trigger cell death by apoptosis. A cancer cell expressing BCL2 is often resistant to apoptosis induced by chemotherapy. This is clearly a selective advantage to the cancer cell, but harmful to the patient.

Multi-step Carcinogenesis and Loss of Heterozygosity

In 1971, Alfred Knudson (Fox-Chase Cancer Center, Philadelphia) described how a deadly childhood cancer, retinoblastoma, requires multiple mutation events to develop. Normally, an individual has two copies of a tumor suppressor gene called RB (for retinoblastoma). Both must be altered for the disease to occur. This is an extremely rare event. Some people are born with one altered copy of the RB gene—that is, they have inherited the mutation. They may live entirely normal lives but pass the affected gene on to their offspring. However, since only one mutagenic "hit" is required to knock out the non-affected gene, they are at much greater risk of developing retinoblastoma. If the offspring of two RB carriers inherits two affected genes, this child will develop the disease without further mutations.

This model applies to other cancers as well. A person who inherits a mutated tumor suppressor gene, needs only one environmental event to knock out the protective effect of its normal allele. A person who has two normal copies of the tumor suppressor gene must sustain two independent mutagenic events in the same cell to initiate a tumor, and therefore has a lower likelihood of developing the disease.

Initiation of cancer often requires a series of mutational events before the normal target cell becomes fully malignant. This process is called transformation. It is thought that at least six mutations must occur for a normal epithelial cell to be transformed to a malignant one. The process usually involves activation of oncogenes as well as inactivation or loss of tumor suppressor genes. In 1991, Bert Vogelstein (Johns Hopkins University, Baltimore) and Ray White (University of Utah, Salt Lake City) independently isolated the APC (adenomatous polyposis colon cancer) gene, which controls the growth of colon epithelium. If this gene is inactivated, a series of mutations follows, leading to development of the disease. This cascade includes activation of certain oncogenes and loss of tumor suppressor genes. Other genes involved in the progression of colon cancer have subsequently been identified and cloned. This concept of multiple mutations leading to cancer, or multi-step carcinogenesis, has been expanded and is now thought to occur in most cancers. The role of multi-step carcinogenesis in breast cancer will be discussed in chapter 4.

An important hallmark of malignant transformation is "loss of heterozygosity" (LOH). Recall that normal cells have two copies of every chromosome and therefore of every gene. Most people are heterozygous at each gene locus, having inherited a particular allele from their mother and another from their father. If DNA is extracted from normal cells and subjected to an analytical process known as agarose gel electrophoresis, the DNA will appear as a series of bands at specific positions in the gel. If an individual is heterozygous at a locus, the two bands for that locus will be at slightly different positions, reflecting the slight differences in their DNA composition. In extracts from cancer cells, one of these bands may be missing. The disappearance of a band often correlates to the loss of a normal tumor suppressor gene. LOH at the p53 locus is especially common in many types of cancers. In sporadic breast cancers, there is often LOH of specific tumor suppressor genes and mutations in the remaining copy, suggesting that the regulatory capability of the gene has been lost.

Relationship Between Mutations and Environmental Factors

Researchers have argued for years whether cancer is caused by faulty genes or by toxins in the environment. In a recent study on 44,788 pairs of twins, some identical and others fraternal, and including two pairs with BRCA2 mutations, Scandinavian investigators concluded that although heritable factors make a minor contribution to susceptibility to most types of cancers, they may have a larger effect on prostate, colorectal, and breast cancers. In their study, 27 percent of breast cancers could be attributed to heritable factors, but the frequency rates of BRCA1 and BRCA2 mutations were too low to explain more than a fraction of the genetic effects observed. The data suggests that defects in other inherited susceptibility genes were involved. The presence of the disease in an identical twin, however, is not a guarantee the other twin will get it. In this study, the risk was 11–18 percent in identical twins, whereas it was only 3–9 percent in fraternal twins and much lower in unrelated subjects. Clearly, genes alone are not the cause of cancer.

Many environmental agents have been implicated in cancer. In our daily lives we are bombarded by potentially dangerous chemicals in our air, water, and food. The news media frequently report that some product or another has been found to cause cancer in laboratory animals. Later they report that the suspected product is really not dangerous to humans, but that another product is potentially dangerous. Likewise, we often hear that eating certain foods or taking certain supplements will protect us from cancer. How do we know what is true? How do we know how to incorporate this information into our lives?

There is no question that our DNA is subject to mutations. Some mutations are repaired or the mutant cell eliminated. Others accumulate until a given cell escapes the normal checks and balances and initiates a tumor. Recall that only a fraction of our DNA serves as genes or regulates gene expression. If the mutation occurs in a non-coding region of DNA or in a cell that is no longer able to divide, it most likely will not have a harmful effect. For a mutation to be dangerous, it must disrupt the function of a regulatory gene in a cell capable of dividing. It also must overcome the effects of its normal allele. Otherwise, the mutation's effect might not be seen.

The actions of certain chemicals and radiation on DNA are so severe that the probability is high that exposure will result in cancer. These types of substances are called complete carcinogens. For example, exposure to ionizing radiation, such as that emitted by the Hiroshima and Nagasaki nuclear blasts or in the Chernobyl disaster, resulted in a high number of cancers among survivors.

Most chemicals that cause mutations require the assistance of other substances, called tumor promoters, to fully transform the damaged cells into malignant tumors. These chemicals are called incomplete carcinogens.

Tumor promoters do not by themselves cause mutations but have the effect of stimulating the cell division that enables mutant cells to propagate. Estrogen and progesterone behave as tumor promoters. Since most mutations require the effects of a promoter to cause cancer, removal of promoters from the environment may help prevent the cancers from developing.

Cancers Related to Specific Mutations (e.g., Retinoblastoma, Ataxia Telangiectasia)

Some cancers are associated with specific gene mutations. I have already mentioned retinoblastoma, which occurs when the tumor suppressing the RB gene is lost or altered. Another disease, ataxia telangiectasia (AT), is caused by a recessive gene. AT patients have increased sensitivity to ionizing radiation and often develop leukemia or lymphoma. Their heterozygous relatives have an increased incidence of breast cancer. There are other cancers associated with inherited defects of specific genes, and some patients with these defective genes also have higher risks of developing breast cancer. These conditions are extremely rare.

Genes Involved with Development and Also with Cancer (Pair Box or Pax Genes)

Normal embryonic development requires precise control of cell division in time and space. Cells divide, differentiate, and migrate according to a precise timetable and map. On a cellular level, the regulation means that transcription of specific genes occurs when the cell is in the proper state of differentiation and in the proper physical environment. The cell receives signals from its environment and those signals are transduced to the nucleus to regulate gene expression. Some of the genes involved in regulating development are also associated with cancer. Among these are PAX, or pair box genes, which were originally identified in the fruit fly but have now been found in many species including human beings. Another developmentally regulated gene is p53, which, if mutated, can be associated with cancer. p53 is discussed in more detail in chapter 4.

4. The Roles of BRCA1, BRCA2, and Other Cancer Genes

The Search for the Breast Cancer Gene

Unlike retinoblastoma or AT, which are caused by a defect in a single gene, breast cancer is multifactorial; it is caused by the interaction of genes and the environment. Most cases are sporadic, occurring in women who have no family history of the disease and no obvious risk factors. At least 30 percent of patients have some family history, however, and 5–10 percent of patients have close relatives with the disease. Clusters of breast cancer cases within an immediate family have been observed for many years. A large study by the National Centers for Disease Control helped identify specific characteristics of inherited breast cancers: Most are diagnosed at an early age (less than forty years old). Many are bilateral, that is, they occur in both breasts. The risk to an individual appears to rise with the number of affected first-degree relatives (mother, daughter, sister). Some patients, or their close relatives, also suffer from ovarian cancer.

Researchers were intrigued by these cases of apparently inherited cancer. They believed the gene causing these cases was dominant and highly penetrant, and sought to locate it and clone it. The competition between investigators eventually became fierce and involved many prominent scientists in the U.S., Canada, Great Britain, and Japan. Researchers including Mary-Claire King (currently at the University of Washington), Francis Collins (National Human Genome Research Institute, National Institutes of Health), Mark Skolnick (Myriad Genetics, Inc.), Bruce Ponder (Cambridge University, United Kingdom), Barbara Weber (University of Pennsylvania), and others were involved in the difficult search. King and Collins initially studied a number of afflicted families and sought to identify specific molecular markers (or identifiable "signposts") on sequences of DNA isolated from white blood cells from these individuals.

If a marker is associated with disease, it suggests that the gene causing the disease is located close to the marker, and that a recombination event between the gene and the marker is not likely to occur. A technique known as linkage analysis tests a battery of markers to find where a specific gene may lie (i.e., by being closely linked to the marker). The strength of the linkage is expressed by a lod score (logarithm of odds). Higher lod scores (three or higher) indicate a high probability of linkage. A lod score of three means that the odds against the linkage occurring by chance are 1,000:1. Distance between markers is measured in centiMorgans (cM), named for the Nobel Prize-winning geneticist Thomas Hunt Morgan. One cM suggests only a 1 percent chance that the markers will separate (recombine) during meiosis (the process of formation of egg and sperm cells). One cM corresponds to approximately one million base pairs of DNA.

The search for a gene involves seeking its specific sequences of A, T, G, and C. Historically it has involved an exhaustive process of screening, sequencing, and excluding candidate genes before the correct one is identified and cloned. A number of technical breakthroughs made in the 1980s and 1990s facilitate localization and identification of specific genes. One of the most significant technical advances has been the development of the polymerase chain reaction (PCR), which permits amplification of small segments of DNA. Another major breakthrough involves the use of restriction fragment length polymorphisms (RFLPs), random variations in DNA sequences, as molecular markers. RFLPs are used in forensics as a DNA "fingerprint" of an individual.

The ultimate goal is to clone the gene being sought. Cloning in this context involves manipulating and growing DNA sequences in bacteria. The technology permits identification of numerous pieces of human DNA, which are archived in genetic "libraries." These so-called cDNA (c is for complementary because they use complementary sequences) libraries permit scientists to determine the linear arrangement of DNA sequences and to create molecular probes for specific sequences. Once a gene is cloned, it is easier to study its role in disease. A full description of the many recent technical advances in molecular biology is beyond the scope of this book. It is important to note, however, that these rapid advances have enabled the Human Genome Project and a private company, Celera, to map almost the entire human genome in about ten years. A "working draft" of the human sequence was produced and published in *Nature* (15 February 2001) simultaneously with a companion publication of the human sequence generated by Celera Genomics Corporation (*Science*, 16 February 2001), identifying the location of perhaps 35,000 genes amidst the three billion base pairs of DNA in each human cell. The work is not yet complete. Human Genome Project is presently focused on completing a finished version of the portions containing most of the genes by spring 2003, two years ahead of the initially projected fifteen-year timetable. The role these genes play can then be elucidated.

Localization of BRCA1 and BRCA2

The hunt for the putative breast cancer genes in the 1980s and early 1990s was far more difficult given the limits of technology available at the time. For example, in the early 1980s, Mary-Claire King worked with a group of twenty-three breast-cancer families (i.e., families who had a number of individuals with breast cancer that were diagnosed before age forty-five). Seventeen showed evidence of genetic linkage to a specific marker on the long arm of chromosome 17, with a lod score of 5.98. This suggests that the likelihood of linkage to a predisposing cancer gene occurring by chance was nearly a million to one. (The other cancer families in this group did not show this linkage, suggesting that they either had a different gene that was responsible for their disease or were exposed to a common environmental agent that caused it.) And yet, the putative cancer gene was still ten cM from the marker, a distance that could encompass as many as five genes.

In 1990, BRCA1 was localized to a position on chromosome 17 (locus 17q21), and it was finally cloned in 1994 by Skolnick's group at Myriad Genetics, Inc., in Salt Lake City.[6] BRCA1 is a large gene consisting of approximately 100,000 base pairs contained in twenty-two exons interspersed by introns and is expressed in breast, ovarian, and some other tissues.

In 1994, Stratton and Goldgar, then at the University of Utah, identified BRCA2, which is localized to chromosome 13 (at 13q12-13) near the RB gene. BRCA1 and BRCA2 gene products normally function as tumor suppressors and repair enzymes.

There are many known mutations of the normal BRCA1 allele. More than 500 BRCA1 sequence variants have been identified. BRCA2 is also subject to numerous mutations. BRCA2 mutations account for most of the hereditary breast cancer not linked to BRCA1, but have less association with ovarian cancer. They are, however, associated with male breast cancer, and possibly prostate, colon, and pancreatic cancers. Mutations of these genes, either by insertion or deletion of non-triplet bases, cause frame shifts that cause transcription of the gene to end prematurely, resulting in truncated proteins that cannot function properly.

Approximately 1–2 percent of Ashkenazi Jewish women have mutations of BRCA1 or BRCA2. In these women, 90–95 percent of the mutations are the same. Two specific mutations (185delAG, a deletion of A and G at position 185, and 538insC, an insertion of C at position 538) affect BRCA1. One mutation (6174delT, deletion of T at position 6174) affects BRCA2 in the Ashkenazi population. Of interest, 2–3 percent of these carry the mutation but have no family history of the disease.

The repeated appearance of a given mutation within a highly inbred population suggests that it is a founder mutation—that is, it occurred in an individual (founder) who then passed it on to progeny where it expanded with the population of descendants. These mutations often begin in small, isolated populations. A genetic bottleneck occurs when the population intermarries. When the population expands again, as did the Ashkenazi Jews in the 17th century, the mutation becomes widespread. The 185delAG mutation in BRCA1 is thought to have occurred forty-six generations ago. The 6174delT mutation in BRCA2 is twenty-nine generations old.

Many mutations of BRCA1 and BRCA2 have been characterized. They are not restricted to the Ashkenazi Jewish community. In fact, 80–85 percent of women with these mutations (which are found in only 0.1–0.3 percent of the general population) are not Ashkenazi Jews. Founder mutations in BRCA1 have also been found in Russia, Sweden, Netherlands, Norway, Scotland, Belgium, and among French Canadians. The highly inbred population of Iceland has a founder mutation in BRCA2 that differs from that found in the Ashkenazi Jewish population. This mutation occurs in a different part of the gene, but the effect is the same: The normal protein coded for by the gene is not synthesized.

Not all carriers of BRCA1 or BRCA2 mutations get cancer. In the Ashkenazi Jewish community, the genes have only 56 percent penetrance. In this population, 16–20 percent of breast cancer patients who develop the disease before age forty have faulty BRCA1 or BRCA2. The penetrance in other communities may be higher, but it is still less than 100 percent. It is still not understood why some people with a given mutation never develop disease while others get it in their thirties. Other co-inherited genetic factors and environmental factors may play a role. Some studies suggest that particular mutations in BRCA1 are more closely associated with ovarian cancer than with breast cancer. In fact, BRCA1 mutations may be involved in as much as 70 percent of familial ovarian cancer but in only 45 percent of familial breast cancer. As many as 10 percent of sporadic ovarian cancers may be due to non-inherited mutations in BRCA1.

Other Breast Cancer Susceptibility Genes

Of the 5–10 percent of breast cancer cases that are inherited, 84 percent are associated with mutations in BRCA1 or BRCA2. The remaining 16 percent are associated with other genes that have not yet been identified but which obviously confer increased susceptibility to disease.

Some genes are associated with cancers of more than one organ or organ system. We have already seen an association between BRCA1 and both breast and ovarian cancers in women. Male breast cancer and some prostate cancers are associated with BRCA2 mutations. A rare condition known as Li-Fraumeni syndrome occurs in families affected by a mutation in the tumor suppressor gene p53, which I introduced in the previous chapter. Normally, the protein product of the p53 gene prevents the cell from entering the S phase of the cell cycle until any damaged DNA is repaired. If DNA is severely damaged, p53 may cause the cell to arrest in G_1, and the cell may undergo apoptosis. If p53 is itself mutated, other damage to the DNA may escape repair, and the altered cell may give rise to cancer. p53 mutations are found in a wide variety of sporadic tumors. It is therefore not unexpected that an inherited p53 mutation would cause a variety of tumors as seen in Li-Fraumeni syndrome. The syndrome is associated with early-onset breast cancer, soft tissue sarcomas, central nervous system tumors, and leukemias. p53 is unusual for a tumor suppressor gene in that it is a dominant negative; inactivation of only one copy of p53 is sufficient to cause cancer.

A number of other, rare cases of genetic predisposition to cancers are correlated with increased risk of breast cancer. Relatives of patients with AT are at higher risk for breast cancer that is not age-dependent. There is also an association between some forms of colon cancer and inherited breast cancer.

Although most cancers are sporadic, chromosomes from the tumor cells show recurrent abnormalities at specific sites. These non-random abnormalities suggest that there are "hot spots" on DNA that are more susceptible to mutations and can be more closely linked to cancer. Many of these sites are associated with known oncogenes or tumor suppressor genes including BRCA1. However, although many chromosomes show non-random abnormalities including oncogene activation or tumor suppressor loss, not all of these changes are associated with specific cancers.

Low-prevalence Risk Genes

In addition to p53 and AT, other genes may contribute to the development of breast cancer. Several "low-prevalence" risk genes are considered to be candidates for "BRCA3," to account for the incidence of familial breast cancer not attributable to BRCA1 or BRCA2 mutations. These risk genes include rare alleles of common genes such as those regulating estrogen or androgen (male hormone) receptors. They also include rare alleles of genes coding for enzymes that are normally involved in detoxifying environmental carcinogens, such as cytochrome P-450, N-acetyl transferase, and gluathione-S-transferase. Abnormalities in these genes, which are normally expressed in breast tissue, may prevent normal detoxification of potentially dangerous substances, resulting in tumor initiation.

It is increasingly apparent that breast cancer is a multifactorial disease, where the interplay of inherited susceptibilities and environmental factors determines who will ultimately develop the disease.

Expression of Specific Genes Associated with Breast Cancer Progression

A number of genes have been identified that are not usually expressed in normal cells but are expressed in cancer cells. Expression of these genes represent pathways that override normal growth controls. A powerful new technology known as DNA microarray analysis permits rapid analysis of gene expression in cancer cells in comparison to normal cells. The use of robotics enables screening of tens of thousands of genes at one time. Recall that the DNA of active genes is transcribed and processed into mRNA. The mRNA can be extracted from cells and, by molecular techniques, transcribed back into DNA. This so-called cDNA differs from the DNA in the cells as all the introns have been excised, and it reflects the genes that are being expressed. cDNAs for many known genes are archived in libraries. To perform DNA microanalysis, small pieces (called oligomers) of DNA derived from cDNA sequences for known genes are embedded onto microchips and incubated with extracts from tumors. Tumor mRNAs hybridize with their cDNA counterparts and can be detected and identified. Since the cDNA sequences embedded on the chips are known, those that hybridize indicate which genes are being expressed in the tumor at that time. Microchips containing sequences of more than 30,000 genes are now commercially available. Tumor extracts can be assessed to determine which of all known genes are turned on and which turned off. The pattern reveals specific molecular pathways utilized by the cancer cells. These profiles give valuable information as to the biology of the tumor. Patterns may differ in different breast cancers and may help distinguish whether the cancer is sporadic or is due to BRCA1 or BRCA2 mutations. The profiles may also be useful in predicting how individual tumors might respond to different therapeutic interventions. To date, DNA microarray technology is being used in research settings, but may soon play an active role in diagnostics and the development of therapies. If a specific molecular pathway can be determined in a given tumor, drugs can be used to inhibit continuing steps in the pathway inhibiting deleterious gene expression.

Some cancer-specific gene products are now used as prognostic indicators because they can mark metastasis or recurrence of disease. Examples include CEA_1, CA15-3, and CA27-29. Elevated levels of these markers in blood are indicators of progressive disease. Some cancer gene products are useful for therapeutic purposes, since antibodies to them can be made. The antibodies can be used to inhibit further growth of malignant cells. Examples include Her2/neu, a shortened version of the epidermal growth factor receptor on normal cells. This gene product is often amplified in breast cancer and has been a marker of an aggressive form of the disease. A new antibody against it (Herceptin) has been showing promise. Another marker, NM23, decreases expression in metastasis and is an indication that the disease is progressing. A cell cycle-dependent tumor suppressor gene product, p16, is associated with 50 percent of breast cancers, and may be a target for future intervention.

It is now apparent that breast cancer, like other cancers, occurs by multi-step carcinogenesis (see chapter 3), requiring alterations in a number of genes. The emerging pattern now suggests that damage to BRCA1 (or a similar tumor suppressor gene) occurs early in ductal epithelial cells. This is followed by LOH of the p53 gene and damage to the remaining copy. The estrogen receptor (ER) gene on chromosome 6 is up-regulated, meaning that more estrogen receptors are expressed on the cells, permitting more estrogen binding and stimulation of growth. In time, there is amplification of the Her2/neu gene as well as others known to play a role in the cell cycle. A decrease of NM23 expression is associated with metastasis. In hereditary breast cancer, the individual is born with one mutated copy of BRCA1 or BRCA2, so that an event that damages the other copy most likely will lead to disease. Since the defect in BRCA genes is inherited in autosomal dominant fashion, a carrier most likely will develop disease. In fact, it is not known if any individuals are homozygous for the BRCA1 or BRCA2 mutations. In sporadic breast cancer, two hits are necessary to initiate the disease, although it is not yet clear that those hits inactivate normal BRCA1 or BRCA2 genes. Mutations in BRCA1 are rarely seen in sporadic breast cancers, and they often differ from those usually seen in inherited BRCA1-related tumors. The hit must occur at a critical codon and alter the amino acid being coded for in order for the mutation to have a phenotypic effect.

Effect of Expression of Hormone Receptors on Breast Cancer Cells

Estrogen and progesterone receptors were discussed in chapter 2. Normal breast tissue cells express receptors for estrogen. Generally, estrogen receptor-positive tumors are less aggressive and are more amenable to hormonal therapy (e.g., tamoxifen). As breast cancers develop, they often show a progressive loss of these receptors. For example, 90 percent of pre-malignant, atypical hyperplasia cells express estrogen receptors, whereas only 50 percent of ductal carcinoma in situ (DCIS) cells and 30 percent of invasive carcinoma cells express them. In post-menopausal women, 75 percent of tumors are likely to be estrogen receptor-positive compared to fewer than 50 percent in younger women, and are often less aggressive.

Tumors associated with BRCA1 mutations tend to be estrogen receptor-negative and less responsive to tamoxifen. However, many of the tumors are medullary carcinoma which tend to be soft and fleshy with scant stroma and usually are not as aggressive as other tumors. BRCA2 tumors tend to be estrogen receptor-positive.

Approximately half of breast cancers are positive for both estrogen and progesterone receptors; 28 percent are negative for both. The remaining tumors are positive for one and negative for the other. In general, patients expressing both estrogen and progesterone receptors on their tumors respond better to hormonal therapy and have a better outcome.

Hereditary vs. Sporadic Breast Cancer: Further Considerations

Although familial breast cancer tends to occur earlier than sporadic and differs histologically, the biology of the two diseases is similar. This observation might suggest that sporadic breast cancer involves random mutations in the same genes that control familial breast cancer. To date, this has not been observed. Statistically, an individual at higher risk of breast cancer due to a known genetic mutation would also be at risk for sporadic breast cancer due to random mutations at another genetic locus. DNA microarray analysis of hereditary and sporadic breast cancer cells may shed light on differences in the two entities. This information could be helpful in determining prognosis and designing therapeutic interventions.

5. Issues in Prevention and Control of Breast Cancer

Understanding Risk

Many women find breast cancer statistics frightening. They often see the "one in eight" statistic in women's magazines and assume they will inevitably get breast cancer. It is no longer considered a matter of "if" but rather "when." Almost everyone knows someone who has been struck by the disease. Ashkenazi Jewish women fear that they have inherited the dreaded breast cancer genes and wonder if they will pass it on to their offspring. Women who know they carry a mutated form of BRCA1 or BRCA2 wrestle with how to prevent what they deem is an inevitable outcome.

I have explained earlier that although the incidence of breast cancer is rising, the statistic one in eight reflects a cumulative or additive risk throughout an individual's lifetime. This type of risk is calculated across the general population, without taking into account ethnic or genetic differences or specific environmental factors that may alter the risk, and is called an absolute risk. Absolute risk is expressed as the number of cases per 100,000 people per year, broken down by age. An individual's risk will probably vary from this ideal risk profile based upon other factors. The absolute risk is like an average risk for a given age. Some individuals will be at higher risk, and others at lower risk, depending upon their specific circumstances. It is similar to the concept of average height in a population. Average height for an American woman might be 5'5", but some will be much taller and others much shorter.

A risk factor is identifiable and makes a person more susceptible to a specific disease. Relative risk compares the incidence of breast cancer in a population with a specific risk factor to that of a reference population without that factor. If the risk of the reference population is one, an individual with a particular risk factor may have a risk of two. This means that the person with the risk factor might be twice as likely to get the disease as the person who does not have the risk factor. However, if at age fifty the reference population has a 2 percent absolute risk of breast cancer, the person with a two-fold relative risk would have a 4 percent chance of contracting it. This is still a low absolute risk. Epidemiologists also refer to attributable risk, which is the amount of disease that could be avoided by eliminating risk factors.

It is important to remember that breast cancer is a multifactorial disease, involving complex interactions between genes and the environment. Some of the apparent risk factors are part of daily living and cannot be avoided. These include being female and getting older. Genetic factors such as ethnic background appear to play a role, as do environmental factors including socioeconomic status.

As I mentioned before, only 5–10 percent of breast cancers can be attributed to a specific, inherited genetic defect such as mutations in BRCA1 or BRCA2, and inheriting these mutations is still not a guarantee that one will develop the disease. A Jewish woman of Ashkenazi descent who has no family history of breast cancer and develops the disease before age fifty has a 13.5 percent chance of having mutations in BRCA1 or BRCA2. A non-Ashkenazi woman with the same family history who develops breast cancer before she is fifty has only an 8 percent chance of having mutations in those genes. An Ashkenazi Jewish woman who develops bilateral breast cancer before age fifty, and who has first- or second-degree relatives with either breast or ovarian cancer diagnosed before age fifty, has a 42–47 percent chance of carrying a mutation in those genes. In contrast, a non-Ashkenazi woman with the same family history who develops breast cancer before age fifty has a 16–33.7 percent risk of having a mutated BRCA gene. Early onset of disease and family history increase the risk that one is carrying the mutated genes, but the disease could still be sporadic.

In 70 percent of breast cancer cases there are no known genetic risk factors. It is of course possible that the incidence of breast cancer in multiple family members could occur by pure chance.

However, 20–25 percent of cases are thought to polygenic: They have a family history of breast cancer, but it cannot be attributed to a single defective gene. These individuals may have inherited a "low prevalence" risk gene. Variant alleles of these genes may confer high sensitivity to ionizing radiation or inefficient detoxification of pesticides or other environmental pollutants. Other gene variants may confer greater sensitivity to estrogen, or predispose to early menstruation or late menopause. A combination of these variant genes and an "appropriate" environmental insult may be necessary to initiate cancer. At least twenty-one genes have already been cloned that are normally involved in the cell cycle as tumor suppressors, proto-oncogenes, or DNA repair enzymes but, upon disruption, may increase susceptibility to cancer.

Modification of Genetic Risk Caused by Environmental Factors

The question arises whether a woman can modify her risk of breast cancer by altering environmental factors that may induce its development. This thinking can apply equally to those who have inherited a faulty gene or to those who are at average risk, since, in either case, environmental factors most likely provide the necessary genetic damage to initiate the onset of disease.

Many potential environmental triggers are still being investigated, and no single culprit has been identified. Different health practitioners offer different suggestions, often reflecting their own particular training and bias. Although scientific studies have been undertaken, many are based on general observations rather than rigorous studies in which experimental data is compared to controlled conditions. Data based upon general observations may show a correlation that does not correspond to cause and effect.

Although female sex hormones are believed to increase the risk for breast cancer, the data is not completely clear. Overall, there appears to be some increased risk if a women begins to menstruate before age twelve, does not have children or has her first child after age thirty, does not breastfeed her children, or undergoes menopause after age fifty-five. The correlation appears to be with the number of ovulatory cycles the woman undergoes in her lifetime. The period between menarche and first pregnancy, during which time the breast tissue is developing, appears to be most sensitive to environmental insults, possibly because rapidly dividing cells have the highest probability of incorporating mutations. It is thought that events initiating breast cancer may occur during this time, but that the promotional events necessary for the disease to be expressed occur over years.

There is interesting evidence from Hiroshima survivors that women exposed to atomic bomb radiation before age twenty had a much higher incidence of breast cancer than those who were in their fifties or older at the time of the attack. The cancers took years to develop, supporting the concept that the developing breasts are more vulnerable to the initial insult, but that promotional events are necessary for the cancer to become apparent. Of course it is possible that those exposed at age fifty did not live long enough afterwards for the tumors to develop. However, atomic bomb survivors were protected from breast cancer by subsequent full-term pregnancies whether they were exposed as children or as adults. Changes occur in the maturation of breast tissue during pregnancy that may be sufficient to reverse early damage that normally would predispose an individual to breast cancer. This observation is in contrast to the fact that breast cancer does occur in pregnant women.

There have been many questions concerning the use of synthetic estrogens as birth control pills or for post-menopausal hormone replacement. It is thought that the estrogens in these preparations increase the risk of breast cancer slightly, but only as consequences of long-term use (i.e., more than ten years). Birth control pills actually decrease the risk of ovarian and endometrial cancer.

Menopausal women with an intact uterus require the addition of progesterone or synthetic progestins to an HRT (hormone replacement therapy) regimen to prevent estrogen-induced endometrial hyperplasia and possibly cancer. For years doctors and scientists believed the drugs caused a slightly elevated risk of breast cancer after long-term use, but conferred protection against cardiovascular disease (heart attacks, strokes, thromboses) and prevented osteo-porosis, the thinning of bones that lead to fractures. HRT was known to prevent uncomfortable symptoms of menopause such as hot flashes, night sweats, mood swings, and vaginal dryness.

The Women's Health Initiative (WHI) is a multi-center study by the National Institutes of Health that focuses on the risks and bene-fits of strategies that could potentially reduce the incidence of heart disease, breast and colorectal cancer, and fractures in post-menopausal women. One of the component clinical trials tested the effects of combined estrogen and synthetic progestin on women with an intact uterus to address the balance of risks and benefits for hormone use in healthy post-menopausal women. 16,608 women between ages fifty and seventy-nine took part in the study, with some receiving the hormone and some receiving a placebo. The trial was stopped abruptly in July 2002, 5.2 years into an eight-year study, due to an increased risk of invasive breast cancer, heart attacks, stroke, and pulmonary embolisms (blood clots) in women taking the hormones. In contrast, the hormone-treated group had fewer fractures and colon cancers. The study was stopped because the risks outweighed the benefits of the combined hormone therapy. Of note, a parallel study using just estrogen in women who had under-gone a hysterectomy did not show an increase in breast cancer, and is still ongoing.

The termination of the WHI study was widely reported and frightened many women. The American College of Obstetricians and Gynecologists (ACOG) urged women not to panic, but to dis-cuss their individual situations with their physicians. Many physi-cians sought guidance on what to tell their patients, but then put the study in perspective: If 10,000 women take the hormone com-bination for one year as compared to 10,000 women not taking the hormone, one would expect to see eight more cases of invasive breast cancer, seven more cases of heart attacks, eight more cases of strokes, and eight more cases of pulmonary embolisms. They would also expect to see six fewer cases of colorectal cancer and five fewer cases of osteoporosis. The increased breast cancer risk did not develop for four years. The increased incidence of pulmonary embolisms occurred in the first two years, and the decrease in colorectal cancer occurred after three years. The increased risks observed applied to an entire population of women, not any individual woman, and did not distinguish between other risk factors a woman might have for breast cancer or other diseases. No distinction was made for ethnic background or the presence of mutations in BRCA1 or BRCA2. ACOG recommends that the decision to stay on hormones or to withdraw be a personal, individualized one based on the woman's individual benefits and risks from such use, but advises that HRT not be used to prevent chronic diseases.

The study utilized a particular combination of conjugated estrogens and the synthetic progestin, medroxyprogesterone acetate, in specific concentrations. Other HRT regimens utilize different formulations of estrogens and progestins or natural progesterone. To date, it is unknown if these formulations would have the same effects. Since the women taking estrogen alone have not shown an increase in breast cancer, the progestins are suspect and will surely be studied further. Recall that progesterone may interact with estrogen to promote potential breast cancers. Of note, women who develop breast cancer while taking hormones often have less aggressive, estrogen-sensitive tumors.

There have been some suggestions that increased dietary fat may predispose a woman to breast cancer. Scientists now believe that total caloric intake and increased weight, as determined by body mass index (BMI), may be a more likely culprit. (BMI is calculated by taking the weight in kilograms and dividing it by height in meters squared.) Estrogen is synthesized in body fat. In an obese post-menopausal woman, this fat may generate sufficient estrogen to promote incipient breast and endometrial cancers. Also, some environmental pollutants are stored in body fat, and may break down and exert estrogen-like effects.

The role of environmental pollutants is hard to assess. Pollutants such as DDT and PCBs are widespread throughout the world and can be found in fish, wildlife, and human tissues including blood and milk. These pollutants have been found in higher concentrations in breast fat of breast cancer patients than in those without cancer. In the absence of epidemiological studies, however, this type of evidence is circumstantial and does not prove a causal relationship. PCBs are organochlorines that are metabolized into weak estrogen-like compounds called xenoestrogens (xeno = foreign). It is not clear if they promote cancer growth. Population studies based on 232 cancer patients and 323 age-matched controls in communities with high rates of breast cancer on Long Island were inconclusive. Similar observations were made in studies on Cape Cod. Studies on cleaning solvents and low-level ionizing radiation such as emitted by power lines and household appliances were likewise inconclusive. To date, no single environmental culprit other than atomic-bomb radiation has been identified, although a combination of environment and predisposing genes will most likely be found to be the cause of most breast cancers.

Role of Diet in Preventing Breast Cancer

We are often bombarded with media reports of dangers in our food supply. There is increased awareness that the ingestion of highly saturated fats and trans-fatty acids is correlated with heart disease if not with cancer. Prepared foods often contain additives that some believe are potentially carcinogenic. There is increased concern about genetically modified corn and other products. Animal feed is often supplemented with antibiotics and hormones that can later be found in meat and milk. Fish and seafood may be contaminated with mercury. Certain methods of cooking meat are believed to generate carcinogens. Nearly every day there is a report that some product or another causes cancer in laboratory animals, although, due to study design requirements for obtaining meaningful data, exposures used are much greater than those ingested by human beings.

There are also reports of specific wholesome and "natural" foods that, if prepared properly and eaten regularly, will prevent cancer. These diets are touted for their purported preventive and even therapeutic effects, and the dietary supplement industry in the United States is booming. These products include vitamins, minerals, trace elements, herbs, and a variety of compounds that are intermediate products of metabolism. We are constantly bombarded by advertisements for products that will protect us against every conceivable illness. What are we to believe?

Most physicians today recommend well-balanced diets that are low in fat and calories and high in fiber, complex carbohydrates, fruits, and vegetables. These foods contain ingredients including antioxidants that may protect DNA from damage by absorbing and inactivating dangerous free radicals that are generated during normal metabolism. They also recommend physical exercise and weight management. Physicians may caution against excessive ingestion of alcohol since there is evidence that alcohol may increase breast cancer risk, especially in women who have no other risk factors. There is no question that physicians will recommend that their patients not smoke, and that they exercise regularly. These recommendations are for an overall healthy lifestyle, not just for prevention of breast cancer.

Many physicians take a guarded view of the benefits of dietary supplements. Since the FDA does not regulate the industry adequately, there are concerns as to the purity of these products, the true concentrations of active ingredients (if they are active), their side effects, and potentially dangerous contaminants. There are also concerns that their actions, if any, may be due to a placebo effect. Specific effects cannot legally be put on labels. Some of these products have potentially dangerous interactions with conventional medicines. Some, however, may be beneficial. For example, most physicians recommend dietary supplements of calcium for perimenopausal and post-menopausal women to help prevent osteoporosis. Soy byproducts known as isoflavones act as phytoestrogens (phyto = plant) and may eliminate some of the discomforts of menopause while not stimulating proliferation of breast tissue.

The sale of these products, however, is driven by economics, not health. The likelihood of diet supplements and modifications in preventing breast cancer is probably small, and they will not cure a tumor that is already growing.

Can Breast Cancer Be Prevented?

Although researchers and clinicians are continuing to learn more about the nature of genetic defects and environmental interactions that may lead to development of breast cancer, no "magic bullet" is currently available for prevention of the disease. In chapter 6 I discuss some of the state-of-the-art research relating to prevention and therapy for the disease. For example, studies have shown that women at high risk can benefit from prophylactic tamoxifen therapy, but there is increased risk of endometrial cancer and potentially fatal blood clots. For now, it will suffice to say that for women of average risk, there are probably no specific options for prevention other than leading an active, healthy lifestyle including exercise and a healthy, well-balanced diet. Some risk factors can be avoided, but involve conscious lifestyle choices. For example, a menopausal woman should carefully weigh the potential risks of classic HRT (breast cancer and cardiovascular disease) versus the benefits of prevention of osteoporosis and colon cancer, and discuss this with her health care provider.

Genetic Testing for BRCA1 and BRCA2: Benefits and Consequences

A woman with a family history of breast cancer and/or ovarian cancer may be facing more difficult questions. Tests are now available for the presence of mutated BRCA1 and BRCA2 genes, but there are many pros and cons to be weighed. There is no correct answer. What works for one woman may not work for another.

The emotional consequences of testing are extremely difficult. Not every woman can handle the knowledge that she has a high probability of developing a potentially deadly disease at an early age. Once a woman learns that she is positive for BRCA1 or BRCA2 mutations, what does she do with that knowledge? Although she is at much higher risk for disease, there is no guarantee that she will actually develop breast or ovarian cancer since the genes are not 100 percent penetrant. These women are still at risk for spontaneous breast cancer (although at a lower risk), as are women with family histories who test negative for the mutated genes.

It is strongly suggested that women who suspect they may have an increased risk of hereditary breast cancer receive genetic counseling. The counselors can help them define and understand their individual risks and recommend possible preventive measures.

The American Cancer Society (ACS) recommends genetic testing if a woman meets any of the following criteria:

- She has more than two first-degree relatives with breast cancer and one with ovarian cancer diagnosed at any age
- She has more than three first-degree relatives diagnosed with breast cancer before age fifty
- She has two sisters diagnosed with breast or ovarian cancer before age fifty
- She has a first-degree relative with two breast cancers, two ovarian cancers, or both breast and ovarian cancer.

A woman with BRCA1 or BRCA2 mutations who develops cancer in one breast has a higher risk of developing it in the other breast as well. Should such a patient have both breasts removed? Some women who have strong family histories of breast cancer elect to undergo prophylactic mastectomies or even oophorectomies (removal of the ovaries) before showing any signs of cancer. Unfortunately, although drastic neither procedure is a guarantee against disease. Sometimes the disease begins and metastasizes so early it is not even detected before surgery, yet can recur years later and be deadly.

Genetic testing raises a major issue as to who has access to sensitive genetic information. Although some laws prevent insurance companies from denying benefits to asymptomatic individuals who take genetic tests, many fear that they will face discrimination in employment or in financial matters such as obtaining loans. The Health Insurance Portability and Accountability Act of 1996 made it illegal for group health plans to consider genetic information a pre-existing condition or to use it to deny or limit coverage. In March 2000, President Clinton issued an executive order banning genetic discrimination in the federal workplace (except for the Department of Defense). (Federal protection for employees against insurance discrimination was already in place.) President Bush also appears to be sympathetic to this issue. States, however, vary in providing protection, and there is no universal mandate for portability. If a woman has genetic tests in a state that offers protection, then moves to another state that does not, she may find herself discriminated against in insurance issues and in the workplace. Since everyone carries perhaps five or six potential disease-related genes, the issue is likely to come before the courts and to garner more media attention in the future.

Chemoprevention

Recent five-year clinical trials of the anti-estrogen compound tamoxifen indicated that chemoprevention may be an effective method of preventing breast cancer in high-risk individuals (including lobular carcinoma in situ, and those with mutated BRCA1 or BRCA2 genes). However, as I indicated above, tamoxifen is not without its own risk. It may lead to endometrial hyperplasia or cancer or cause thromboses. It also causes temporary premature menopause, with all the associated discomforts, and some patients develop resistance to the drug. New studies are under way comparing tamoxifen to a similar drug, raloxifene (Evista®), that may have similar beneficial effects with fewer side effects.

Importance of Early Detection

Although the incidence of breast cancer is increasing, its death rate has been steady since 1990 and may even be dropping. Much of this increased survival can be attributed to increased awareness leading to early detection of the disease, and treating it before it has had a chance to spread. The importance of early detection cannot be stressed enough, whether or not a woman has a family history of the disease.

Early detection can be achieved by monthly breast self-examination. The American Cancer Society publishes pamphlets and shower cards to demonstrate the procedure. Although noted breast surgeon Dr. Susan Love recommends that this exam not be limited to once per month, other physicians feel that it should be done just after a woman's menstrual period, or on a given day of the month for women who are no longer menstruating, so that women get into the habit of regular self-exams. Most health-care practitioners would agree with Dr. Love that women should get to know their own breasts, and to recognize what is normal and what is not. Furthermore, a woman should have her breasts examined at least once per year by a competent health care practitioner.

Although there have been reports of new diagnostic tests, mammography remains the best screening technology available today. The newest mammography machines deliver minimal X-ray radiation and permit the trained radiologist to detect lesions as small as 0.5 centimeters (0.2 inches) (fig. 5.1). New digital imaging technology is further improving the detection of tiny lesions, especially in the presence of dense breast tissue. The American Cancer Society guidelines currently recommend that a baseline mammogram be done at forty years of age, then repeated every two years until age fifty. The American College of Radiology, however, believes that clinical trials have shown that by having screening mammograms every year, compared to every one to two years for women in their forties, breast cancers are found at an earlier stage. The earlier breast cancers are detected, the better are the chances for good treatment results. All agree that after age fifty, the test should be repeated

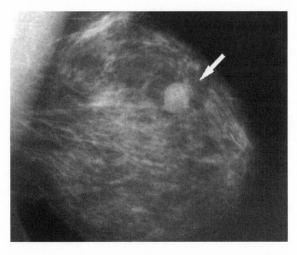

Fig. 5.1 A small breast cancer (arrow) detected by mammography. The tiny white spots are benign microcalcification.

annually. The benefit of mammography in younger women is more limited due to the high density of their breast tissue. Also, since the effects of ionizing radiation such as X-ray are cumulative, many physicians feel it is unwise to expose younger women to even this limited amount.

A recently reported Danish study questions whether mammography truly increases survival of breast cancer patients. The study has garnered much media attention and will be the subject of a Congressional inquiry. However, the American Cancer Society has stayed firm in its mammography guidelines and recommendations, and a recent Swedish study found a clear survival benefit for those having regular mammograms.

Some women hesitate to have mammograms for fear of discomfort or of learning that they actually do have breast cancer. Mammograms may not be comfortable, but they are rarely painful and they do not take very long. The discomfort involved is certainly worthwhile, considering that the result of avoiding the test could be the difference of life or death.

Some other diagnostic tools that have been written about in popular publications include ultrasound, MRI (magnetic resonance imaging), CT (computerized tomography) scans, and PET (positron emission tomography) scans. Ultrasound is of value in distinguishing between a fluid-filled cyst and a solid lump. MRI, CT, and PET scans may be helpful in detecting the spread of breast cancer to internal organs or recurrence of a previously diagnosed cancer. However, none of these techniques has proven as valuable as mammography for early detection of a potential cancer within the breast.

What Happens If You Find a Lump: Diagnostic Procedures

A woman will most often find a lump or other abnormality while doing self-examination of her breasts. A majority of these lumps are not cancer, but it is imperative that a health care practitioner be consulted as soon as possible. The physician will most likely want to perform a clinical breast exam. Depending upon those findings, the patient may be sent to obtain a diagnostic mammogram.

Occasionally a man will discover a lump in his chest in the area of the nipple. He too should have a medical consultation, even though breast cancer in men is rare. If diagnosed late, it can be as deadly as in women. The risk in males is higher if they have a family history of BRCA2-associated disease. A male may also be referred for mammography.

Since a mammogram can detect a tumor that is 0.5 cm (0.2 inches), it can detect one that is not yet palpable. Tumors are rarely palpable if they are less than 0.4 inches in diameter. The presence of microcalcifications raises the index of suspicion, although they are not always associated with cancer. When widespread, they may just reflect normal "wear and tear." The radiologist may request additional enhancement views, and will compare the current mammogram to those taken in previous years. The patient may also be referred for an ultrasound to distinguish between fluid-filled cysts and solid tumors.

Suspicious lumps are diagnosed by biopsies. The specific type of biopsy depends upon the nature of the mass as well as its location. The simplest biopsies are done through special hollow needles. Fluid that contains cells may be aspirated, or a core of tissue may be removed. Incisional or excisional biopsies are full surgical procedures in which a surgeon removes samples of the tumor or the entire tumor and sends them to a pathologist for examination. Surgical biopsies are usually done in outpatient facilities, usually under local anesthesia.

Current Treatments for Breast Cancer

If the lesion proves to be malignant, there is now a wide variety of treatment options. This book is intended to be a general guide, but new treatment protocols are constantly being developed. Different medical centers use different experimental and standard treatment protocols. Remember that every breast cancer is unique. The best option for a given patient is a matter for the patient and the health care provider.

Today, patients are usually informed of their options and are given choices. Although it is important not to delay, they are usually given some time to think about the options and to arrive at decisions with which they and their loved ones are comfortable. In major medical centers, patients are often treated by a multidisciplinary team that may include a surgeon, radiation oncologist, medical oncologist, radiologist, pathologist, nurse practitioner, and social worker. Most traditional treatments for breast cancer involve some combination of surgery, chemotherapy, and/or radiation. However, the extent of surgery and subsequent therapy depend upon the nature of the tumor and whether it has spread to lymph nodes or beyond. Oncologists refer to the grade and stage of cancers, where grade reflects morphologic (structural) abnormalities in the cells themselves, and stage refers to the size of the tumor and how far it has spread. Higher grades and stages are often associated with worse prognoses (table 5.1). Breast cancer treatment guidelines published by the National Comprehensive Cancer Network (NCCN) and the American Cancer Society (ACS) are summarized in table 5.2. These guidelines were updated in June 2000 and are the most current available.

Table 5.1 Staging of Breast Cancers. Breast cancers are staged according to a combination of criteria known as the TNM system

Stage	T	N	M
0	Lobular carcinoma in situ or ductal carcinoma in situ		
I	0–2 cm	0	0
II	0–2 cm	1+	0
	2–5 cm	0 or 1+	0
IIIA	5+ cm	1+	0
	Fixed or ulcerated	0 or 1+	0
IIIB	Any size	Large or near collarbone	0
	Spread to skin, chest wall, or internal mammary nodes		
IV	Any size	0 or 1+	1+ sites

T stands for the size of the tumor (in centimeters), whether it is fixed to the skin or to underlying muscle, and whether it has ulcerated. N stands for whether or not the lymph nodes are positive, and if so, their size, and where they are located. M stands for whether or not the tumor has metastasized (spread) to other locations. Staging is often used to determine the best course of treatment for a patient. The lower the stage, the better the prognosis. Notice that there are several possible combinations for stages II and III. (Adapted from Susan M. Love with Karen Lindsey, *Dr. Susan Love's Breast Book,* 3rd ed. Perseus Publishing, 2000 and joint publication of the American Cancer Society (ACS) and National Comprehensive Cancer Network (NCCN). <http://www.cancer.org/downloads/CRI/breast_cancer_guidelines.pdf> (2000).)

Table 5.2 Current breast cancer treatment guidelines			
Stage	**Surgery**	**Radiation**	**Chemotherapy**
0 (LCIS)	NO (just close observation for most women)	NO	Tamoxifen
0 (DCIS)	1 quadrant affected – lumpectomy or	YES	Tamoxifen
	mastectomy	NO	Tamoxifen
	2+ quadrants – mastectomy	NO	Tamoxifen
I & II	Lumpectomy and node biopsy or	YES	Maybe
	Modified radical mastectomy	YES 4+ nodes + NO if small and node -	YES
III	Lumpectomy or mastectomy and node dissection	YES	YES
IV	Rare to present with Stage IV; If had prior lumpectomy, do mastectomy	NO	Hormonal therapy Chemotherapy Herceptin Taxol Palliative support

These guidelines are general. Specific treatment depends upon many factors, including the pathology report of the initial biopsy (i.e., type of tumor); whether or not the patient is pre- or post-menopausal, presence or absence of estrogen/progesterone receptors; presence or absence of Her2/neu; results of scans for metastasis; and whether or not the tumor has recurred. Of note, no reference is made if the patient is BRCA1 or BRCA2 positive. (Adapted from a joint publication of the American Cancer Society (ACS) and National Comprehensive Cancer Network (NCCN). <http://www.cancer.org/downloads/CRI/breast_cancer_guidelines.pdf> (2000).)

In chapter 3 I discussed the pattern of breast cancer invasion and dissemination through the body via the lymphatics. Some breast surgeons prefer to dissect and examine the nodes under the armpit. Prognosis may depend upon whether or not the nodes are involved with disease, and if so, how many are. Some surgeons employ a fairly new technique called a sentinel lymph node biopsy. A blue dye or a radioactive substance is injected into the tumor. The dye drains into the sentinel node, i.e., the first lymph node into which the tumor drains and the one most likely to contain cancer cells if the tumor has spread. The surgeon can see the blue dye in the sentinel node or can detect the radioactivity with a Geiger counter. This node is removed and examined for the presence of tumor cells. If it is negative, subsequent nodes are likely to be negative, and the cancer has most likely not spread. The patient can avoid the risks and discomfort of a full node dissection, especially that of lymphedema, in which lymph fluid causes swelling and pain in the affected arm and hand. However, if the sentinel node is positive, a full lymph node dissection is usually indicated.

The tumor cells are evaluated for hormone receptors and other cell surface receptors (markers) such as Her2/neu that may influence the course of treatment.

Other diagnostic tests may include routine blood analysis to see if there is evidence of anemia or abnormal blood chemistries. These tests may indicate involvement of the bone marrow and the bones themselves with tumor. The tumor's S-phase fraction (SPF), or percentage of tumor cells replicating DNA, gives an indication of how fast a tumor is growing. A Ki-67 test identifies cells in S-phase as well as cells preparing to replicate DNA, cells that have completed DNA replication, and cells in the process of dividing.

Treatment of Breast Cancer

Depending upon the nature of the particular tumor, a surgeon may elect to do a lumpectomy in which the tumor and a wide margin of normal surrounding tissue is removed, or to do a total mastectomy in which the entire breast is removed. The disfiguring Halstead radical mastectomy, in which the muscle of the chest wall is also removed, is rarely done today. The patient is usually involved in the decision-making process. Most surgeons attempt to spare as much breast tissue as possible (breast conserving surgery), and are sensitive to the cosmetic issues involved. Insurance companies today pay for reconstructive plastic surgery if the patient is a candidate for such a procedure.

Surgery is usually followed by an additional (adjuvant) therapy. A lumpectomy is usually followed by a course of radiation to destroy undetected cancer cells that may have been left behind in the breast, chest wall, or lymph nodes and that have the potential to metastasize. Some lumpectomy and most mastectomy patients also receive chemotherapy in which toxic drugs are given orally or by IV to block DNA synthesis or division of cancer cells (table 5.3). Although the drugs target tumor cells, they are not specific and affect all rapidly dividing cells such as those in hair follicles, intestinal lining, and bone marrow. That is why chemotherapy causes such unpleasant side effects as hair loss, vomiting, and low blood cell counts. Chemotherapy may also cause premature menopause and infertility. Chemotherapy is usually given in cycles, with each period of treatment followed by a period of recovery. The total course of treatment can span three to six months. Side effects usually vary with the specific drugs used, their dosages, and duration of treatment. There are now drugs available that prevent or reduce the nausea and vomiting. There are also new drugs called growth factors that help the bone marrow recover, speeding up the recovery of red and white blood cell counts and thereby improving blood counts. Platelets, however, if needed, must be transfused, and patients receive antibiotics to counteract the high risk of infection.

Different chemotherapy drugs inhibit DNA synthesis or cell division by different mechanisms. Some inhibit both DNA and RNA synthesis. Others stop the process of mitosis. The drugs are often given in combination, following standard protocols. Since tumor cells usually have many genetic aberrations that favor uncontrolled growth, these protocols are designed to hit the tumor cells in multiple ways. Combination chemotherapy also helps protect against the development of resistance to a single drug.

Drug resistance often develops when mutated cells amplify (increase the number of copies of) genes for transporter molecules such as p-glycoprotein. These molecules bind to the drug and transport it out of the cell before it can do damage. This

Table 5.3 Examples of chemotherapy agents and combination protocols			
Generic Name	**Brand Name**	**Method of Action**	**When Used**
Cyclophosphamide	Cytoxan	Interferes with tumor growth	primary and metastatic
Doxirubicin	Adriamycin	Inhibits DNA synthesis	primary and metastatic
Epirubicin	Ellence	Inhibits DNA synthesis	primary and metastatic
5-Fluorouracil	5-FU	Inhibits DNA and RNA synthesis	primary and metastatic
Methotrexate		Interferes with DNA synthesis and repair	primary and metastatic
Docetaxel	Taxotere	Inhibits cell division	"rescue therapy" after failure of first chemo
Etoposide	VePesid	Stops cell division	metastatic
Mitoxantrone	Novantrone	Inhibits DNA synthesis	metastatic
Mitomycin C	Mutamycin	Inhibits DNA synthesis	metastatic
Paclitaxel	Taxol	Inhibits cell division	metastatic
Vinblastine	Velban	Inhibits cell division	metastatic
Vinorelbine	Navelbine	Inhibits cell division	metastatic
Capecitabline	Xeloda	Converts to 5-FU	resistant metastatic
Trastuzumab	Herceptin	Blocks Her2/neu	metastatic with Her2/neu over-expression (excessive amount of Her2/neu protein on cell surfaces)

(Adapted from Susan M. Love with Karen Lindsey, *Dr. Susan Love's Breast Book,* 3rd ed. Perseus Publishing, 2000 and joint publication of the American Cancer Society (ACS) and National Comprehensive Cancer Network (NCCN). <http:www2.cancer.org/nccn_acs/ breast/> (1999).)

(*continued*)

Table 5.3 (*continued*)	
Common Combined Chemotherapy Protocols	
Protocol Name	**Drugs Used**
CMF	Cyclophosphamide (Cytoxan), Methotrexate, and Fluorouracil
CAF	Cyclophosphamide, Doxorubicin (Adriamycin), and Fluorouracil
AC	Adriamycin, Cyclophosphamide +/− Paclitaxel (Taxol)
A + CMF	Adriamycin followed by CMF

phenomenon is called multiple drug resistance. Another mechanism of resistance is the expression of BCL2 in cancer cells, preventing apoptosis that would normally be induced by radiation or chemotherapy.

Sometimes, chemotherapy is given prior to surgery (neo-adjuvant therapy) for the purpose of shrinking the tumor to make it more amenable to surgical removal. Tiny lesions, less than 1.0 cm in size and without lymph node involvement, may not require adjuvant therapy. The details depend upon the specific patient and the nature of the disease.

In addition to conventional chemotherapy, some patients are treated with hormone or antibody therapy. Those expressing estrogen and/or progesterone receptors (ER-positive and PR-positive) more likely will respond to hormone treatment. Patients with ER-positive tumors may do well with tamoxifen or another anti-estrogen treatment. Tamoxifen may also benefit patients whose tumors are ER-negative, especially if they are PR-positive. Since the expression of progesterone receptors is regulated by estrogen receptors, tamoxifen may bind to estrogen receptors that are below the threshold for detection yet may still exert an effect. Treatment with tamoxifen for five years after the initial surgery has reduced breast cancer recurrence by 42 percent and mortality by 22 percent. However, the treatment induces premature menopause in

Table 5.4 Examples of hormonal therapy agents			
Generic Name	**Brand Name**	**Method of Action**	**When Used**
Anastrozole	Arimidex	Aromatase inhibitor [prevents estrogen synthesis]	Post-menopausal women who failed on Tamoxifen
Exemestrone	Aromasin	Aromatase inhibitor	Advanced disease; post-menopausal; ER+
Goserelin	Zoladex	Blocks FSH/LH	Advanced disease; pre-menopausal
Letrozole	Femara	Aromatase inhibitor	Advanced disease; post-menopausal; ER+
Megestrol Acetate	Megace	Unclear	Advanced disease; progression after Tamoxifen
Tamoxifen	Nolvadex	SERM [blocks estrogen in breast, not uterus]	Breast cancer prevention; primary and metastatic disease
Toremifene citrate	Fareston	SERM anti-estrogen	Metastatic disease; post-menopausal; ER+

(Adapted from Susan M. Love with Karen Lindsey, *Dr. Susan Love's Breast Book,* 3rd ed. Perseus Publishing, 2000.)

perimenopausal women, and may increase the risk of uterine cancer and thromboses. Patients with hormone receptor-positive tumors may also be treated with aromatase inhibitors that block the production of estrogen. A list of hormonal therapies is presented in table 5.4.

Tumors expressing high levels of Her2/neu tend to be exceptionally fast growing and aggressive. These patients may receive antibody therapy with Herceptin (trastuzumab). Response to this treatment is promising. These tumors often respond to certain chemotherapy protocols as well.

Bone marrow and/or stem cell transplantation for metastatic breast cancer has not been as successful as hoped, but procedures are improving and the therapy is still being evaluated in clinical trials. The treatment is generally used in patients with advanced disease or with a high risk of recurrence. The principle of this treatment is to remove the blood-producing stem cells from the bone marrow or peripheral circulation of the patient, remove any trace of cancer cells, and store them. The patient is then subjected to high dose chemotherapy and/or radiation to kill tumor cells that have metastasized throughout the body and are not amenable to surgical excision. This high level of chemotherapy and/or radiation destroys the rapidly dividing cells of the marrow, including the crucial stem cells. Without these stem cells, the patient would be unable to produce white cells to fight infection, red cells to carry oxygen, or platelets to prevent excessive bleeding. Following chemotherapy, the patient's stored stem cells are then reinfused in the hope that they will engraft and reconstitute the immune system. Unfortunately, the procedure still has a high mortality rate, and it is questionable if it extends life or even improves the quality of life for breast cancer patients.

Breast cancer patients are usually followed carefully to check for recurrences. Despite early diagnosis and aggressive therapy, breast cancer may recur, often within two years. The recurrence may be local, at the site of the original tumor, or it may affect lymph nodes and distant sites such as lung, liver, bones, and brain. Worrisome signs include new lumps at the site of the original tumor, pain in spine and hips, cough and respiratory difficulties, headaches and loss of balance, and unexplained weight loss. Diagnostic tests such as bone scans help identify the site of recurrences. Recurrent breast cancers may require additional surgery and more aggressive chemotherapy, but do not necessarily pronounce a death sentence. In patients with advanced disease, however, the treatment options are more limited. End stage disease is marked by widespread metastases to vital organs. For these patients, the recommended therapies are focused on pain management and nutritional support.

A current "hot topic" concerns the treatment of ductal carcinoma in situ (DCIS). These tumors are malignant but are confined to the duct, and so are not yet considered invasive carcinomas. They are often detected by mammography when they are tiny. The question arises as to how vigorously they should be treated. Breast cancer specialists are learning that some tiny tumors may have invasive potential, while larger tumors may grow slowly and never invade. It is hoped that information gleaned from DNA microarray technology will elucidate the biological differences of these tumors so that the most conservative treatments can be safely applied in a given situation. In the meantime, patients are advised to make their decisions together with their health care providers. New treatments are currently being developed that aim to spare patients from the miseries of extensive surgery, radiation, and/or chemotherapy.

Clinical Trials

Clinical trials are studies in which a promising new drug or experimental treatment is tested on a group of people. Researchers try to assess whether this treatment works better than others already available, what side effects it produces, whether the benefits outweigh the risks (including side effects), and which patients will most likely be helped. The drug will have already been tested extensively in animals. Groups of patients are randomly assigned to receive either a drug being tested or standard treatment. The studies are often double-blind—that is, neither the patient nor the researcher knows who is receiving the experimental drug and who is receiving the standard one.

Phase I trials test the safety, side effects, and safe dosage ranges of the drug. It is tested on a small group of people (twenty to eighty). Phase II trials test whether the drug is safe and effective on a larger group of people (100–300). They may also test the best way to give the drug to the patient. Phase III trials, conducted on 1,000–3,000 people, compare the results of this drug with the standard treatment and monitor its side effects. The researchers can compare the two treatments and determine whether the new treatment is better for survival and quality of life. They may measure whether the growth of the cancer slows and how long the patients remain disease-free. Side effects are carefully monitored at each phase, and the trial is discontinued if the side effects are too severe.

Clinical trials have specific guidelines and inclusion/exclusion criteria for patients who wish to participate. These criteria are based on many factors that insure the quality of the trial and that keep participants safe. A patient interested in enrolling usually discusses the possibility with his or her physician, and then contacts the study's research staff about a particular trial.

Patients who enroll in clinical trials have no guarantee that they will receive the treatment being tested rather than an older one. The patients must give full informed consent, and are free to withdraw from the study at any time. Participation in a clinical trial may not benefit a given patient but may be of value to others in the future. It is important for patient and physician to clearly understand the benefits and pitfalls of participating in a clinical trial. More information on clinical trials is presented in the appendix.

Considerations for "Alternative" Medicine

Some patients choose to obtain care from practitioners of "alternative" medicine. They may consult naturopaths, homeopaths, or herbologists, and are treated with assorted diets and herbal therapies. None of these, however, has ever been tested on breast cancer in a clinical trial, nor is there any credible evidence of their effectiveness. Furthermore, some unproven treatments can interfere with standard medical treatments or may cause serious side effects. Nevertheless, alternative medicine is becoming so popular in the United States that some medical schools are beginning to discuss its use as adjuncts to evidence-based treatments. Co-treatments by practitioners of alternative medicine may offer some comfort to patients who are terminally ill. However, most scientifically trained physicians do not recommend these treatments as alternatives to established protocols.

Potentials for Gene Therapy

The protocols for treating breast cancer do not differ between patients with hereditary or spontaneous disease, since the diseases are not different. Much attention has been placed on Human Genome Project discoveries and the possibilities of gene therapy. Patients with known BRCA1 or BRCA2 mutations wonder whether these defective genes can be corrected by such treatment. While gene therapy is perceived as a treatment of the future, current experience is a "mixed bag." It is especially difficult to address issues of germ-line mutations (which BRCA mutations are) given the current controversy and restrictions on embryonic stem cell or fetal tissue research. I address this issue in greater detail in chapter 6.

The Need for Emotional Support

Physicians and others who care for breast cancer patients are becoming more sensitive to quality-of-life issues. An important part of breast cancer therapy is emotional support both for the patient and for the family. Many women feel a deep sense of loss following mastectomy and even lumpectomy, and need the support that can be provided by professional counselors. Chemotherapy often causes hair loss, induces premature menopause, and may cause serious mood swings that affect not only the patient but also her loved ones. Many medical centers now provide integrated services including physicians, surgeons, nutritionists, and social workers as part of a team. Patients often have supportive family members and friends, or may be part of a religious group or other organization that provides support sessions and religious "healing" services. A diagnosis of cancer is a life-altering event even if the prognosis for long-term survival is excellent.

Some patients and their families even find a positive side to their ordeal—the realization that every day is a special gift to be savored and lived to the fullest. An individual patient's reaction is highly variable, but all need support. For those who are terminally ill, the services of a hospice may provide relief from pain and a place to die in dignity. A list of resources for information and support is provided in the appendix.

6. Breast Cancer Research

A major research focus has been to understand the events that initiate the disease at the molecular and genetic level. The ultimate goal is to develop strategies to prevent the disease from occurring. Alternatively, molecular and genetic information can be utilized in the development of new therapies to treat, cure, or at least to control the disease, while eliminating some of the debilitating side effects that are associated with current cancer treatment.

The Search for More Predisposing Genes

The discovery of BRCA1 and BRCA2 has launched a new era in the quest to understand the causes of breast cancer. Now that the human genome has been mapped, the focus of molecular biologists will be on understanding the role of the approximately 35,000 genes that define a human being. A new field of proteomics is being developed in which the role of gene-encoded proteins is studied. Already, the dogma that one gene encodes a single protein is not certain. The gene encodes the primary backbone of the protein, but other factors control the processing that makes the three-dimensional, functional molecule and regulates how the molecule functions in the cell.

There are many questions concerning genetic intervention in multifactorial diseases such as breast cancer. We already know that BRCA1 and BRCA2 do not account for all the cases of hereditary breast cancer, and that the disease is influenced by other genes and environmental factors. It is likely that, in coming years, other predisposing genes and their protein products will be elucidated. The interaction of these with environmental agents will be further examined in an effort to understand why the genes become damaged, why certain regions of genes are "hot spots" for mutations, and why the damage results in cancer.

The Role of Cross-talk Between Malignant Cells and Their Surroundings

A focus of current research is to understand how a malignant cell's environment modifies its behavior. This approach is called epigenetic, because the target is not the gene itself but rather factors that regulate the expression of the gene. A gene may be damaged, but its expression may be controlled so that its altered product may not be produced. In other words, cancer may be preventable if we can change the environment the gene acts on rather than changing the genetically altered cell. For example, researchers have focused on the role of genetic damage in the ductal cells in initiating breast cancer, but the role of the surrounding stromal cells has been more or less ignored. It is now increasingly apparent that there is cross-talk between the ductal cells, where breast cancer usually begins, and surrounding cells, and that the stroma may play a role in preventing carcinoma in situ from breaking through into an invasive cancer. It has also been postulated that specialized epithelial cells that surround the ducts may secrete an enzyme that can control the emergence of invasive carcinoma. Epigenetic events may also explain tumor dormancy, in which metastatic cancers recur many years after the primary tumor has been diagnosed and treated. What causes these silent tumors to reemerge and resume their rampage? Understanding epigenetic phenomena may enable us to control cancer if not cure it. In this context, pre-cancerous conditions such as atypical hyperplasia could possibly be reversed, thereby avoiding the development of a true cancer.

Most research is being done in animal models or in cultured tumor cells. While we may now recognize the earliest pre-malignant changes that occur in isolated ductal cells, we do not yet have diagnostic tests than can detect those changes. Some research is directed toward developing more sensitive, non-invasive imaging. One possible screening procedure is somewhat analogous to the familiar Pap smear for cervical cancer (named for Dr. Papanicolaou, who developed the technique). The method is called breast ductal lavage, in which saline is introduced into individual ducts in the nipples and then extracted. Some ductal cells slough off and are found in the extracted fluid. The presence of atypical cells may be a warning of incipient cancer and early treatment may reverse the process. However, since there are from five to nine ductal systems in each breast, and the procedure is fairly uncomfortable, it is not widely used.

Diagnostics

Diagnostic imaging techniques are intended to identify tumors at the earliest possible stages. Ultimately, the goal is to distinguish between dense tissue, benign lumps, and cancer. To date, mammograms still offer the best imaging available for early diagnosis of breast cancer. However, they are not foolproof, and miss perhaps 10 percent of cancers. In younger women with dense breast tissue, mammograms may not distinguish a small tumor from surrounding tissue, although digital enhancing may enhance the sensitivity. They often cannot detect lobular carcinoma in situ in early stages. They are not reliable in women who have breast implants, nor do they distinguish fluid-filled cysts from solid fibroadenomas as well as does ultrasound. Current research is focused on better imaging with the least possible radiation.

Other imaging techniques such as MRI, PET scans, MIBI (nuclear medicine) scans, and thermography have more limited diagnostic applications. CT scans generate too much radiation to be used safely for breast tissue.

Therapeutics

Cancer therapy, including that for breast cancer, has traditionally taken a "slash, poison, and burn," approach where the tumor is subjected to surgical eradication, followed by chemotherapy and radiation to remove any malignant cells that may remain. Although this aggressive approach is still used, efforts are made to use the most conservative surgery possible (including options for breast reconstruction where possible), chemotherapy protocols based on increased knowledge of the biology of the disease, and radiation that targets the tumor but as little normal tissue as possible.

Chemotherapy for cancer generally employs chemicals that poison all rapidly growing cells. New knowledge of the molecular and genetic bases for cancer is enabling the development of drugs that target cancer cells more specifically, thereby eliminating some of the side effects. An example of molecular based therapy is Herceptin, the new antibody against the Her2/neu receptor. Her2/neu is expressed in 70 percent of DCIS, but only in 30 percent of invasive cancers. In metastatic breast cancers, the receptor is often over-expressed or has too many copies of itself on cell surfaces due to too many copies of the gene. Metastatic cancers over-expressing Her2/neu tend to be particularly aggressive, but are showing a good response to Herceptin. The antibody binds specifically to these cells and causes the cells to stop dividing. Furthermore, for reasons not yet understood, patients who respond to Herceptin are also more likely to respond to certain chemotherapy agents than to others.

Research is continuing into the properties of different estrogen receptors (chapter 2). These properties have led to the development of such selective estrogen receptor modulators (SERMs) as tamoxifen and raloxifene. New drugs are being developed to further exploit the properties of these receptors and the signals they send to the cell's nucleus to modulate gene expression.

The effects of natural progesterone and synthetic progestins are also being studied in terms of their binding to different classes of receptors and differences in the signaling pathways that follow. Dr. Kathryn Horwitz's laboratory at the University of Colorado Health Sciences Center is studying the complex interaction of estrogen, progesterone, growth factors, and cytokines in breast cancer. Whereas progesterone alone causes cell-cycle arrest in isolated breast cancer cells and confers protection against estrogen-induced endometrial hyperplasia in the uterus, progesterone in combination with estrogen induces breast tissue proliferation in vivo. It also has effects on many signal transduction pathways that stimulate cell growth.

Progesterone binds to two naturally occurring receptors, PR-A and PR-B, that are functionally distinctive mediators of progesterone action. Mice that lack PR-A develop mammary glands, but do not counteract the proliferative effect of estrogen on the uterine endometrium and do not have normal reproductive functions. PR-A is therefore involved in anti-estrogen and anti-proliferative activity in the uterus and normal reproduction. Mice lacking PR-B do not develop mammary glands but reproduce normally. The different tissue-specific signaling pathways of PR-A and PR-B are being studied in the hope of designing a progestin-based hormone replacement or therapeutic drug that protects both the breast and uterus from proliferative effects of estrogen.

Recall that multiple events must occur before a damaged cell becomes malignant, and before a localized cancer becomes a dangerous, metastatic disease. The particular chain of events may be regulated by a variety of factors including the expression of susceptibility genes, the nature of the carcinogen(s), and the immunologic status of the patient. Genetic and epigenetic factors determine why one patient exposed to the same environmental insult gets cancer and another does not. Dr. Anthony Elias at the University of Colorado Health Sciences Center is conducting studies to define these molecular pathways for the progression of disease and to predict recurrence. The new DNA microarray technology is greatly assisting this endeavor. Already it is apparent that pathways utilized by one class of cells (e.g., estrogen receptor–positive) differ from those of another class (e.g., estrogen receptor–negative). The patterns of gene expression correlate to the protein surface markers exhibited by specific types of breast cancer cells. These markers have been hallmarks of pathologists' diagnoses for years. Elucidation of these biochemical pathways will help researchers determine the biological potential of the cells (e.g., growth rates, metastatic potential) and help identify more precisely who is at risk for aggressive disease so that the patient can be treated accordingly.

As scientists learn more about the regulation of gene expression in cancer cells, new drugs can be specifically designed to block steps in those pathways. New drugs being tested include those that may act epigenetically to control the altered cell's microenvironment. Among candidates are thalidomide, which prevents growth of blood vessels to the tumor, and certain anti-inflammatory drugs such as cyclooxygenase-2 inhibitors. Other drugs specifically target the cancer cells. Tamoxifen binds competitively with estrogen to estrogen receptors so cancer cells dependent upon the hormone cannot grow. Herceptin binds to the Her2/neu receptor expressed by certain cancer cells and kills the cells expressing the receptor but not normal cells, thereby minimizing side effects.

Gene Therapy

Elucidation of the genes involved in breast cancer is prompting continued research in gene therapy. The goal of gene therapy is to replace the defective gene with a normal one or to counteract its expression, and thereby prevent the inherited disease from occurring. Other gene therapy approaches target cancer cells with a lethal gene that will kill just the malignant cells but not normal surrounding cells. There have been some success stories with this approach in conditions caused by single gene defect. There have also been failures, including a well-publicized case in which a young man died during experimental gene therapy that was not clinically necessary. Many of the problems of gene therapy involve the delivery of the target genes to the site in which they must act. The gene is carried in a vector that must seek out only the correct target. This is especially difficult to achieve in a heterogeneous, metastatic cancer. A recent study targeted elements in the stroma of a tumor rather than the cancer cells themselves. The vector accumulated in the tumor, transferred lethal genes to the tumor cells and killed them while sparing non-dividing cells. In multifactorial diseases such as breast cancer, where penetrance of even a known susceptibility gene is not complete, it is hard to devise a strategy for a gene-based therapeutic approach. Some experiments are under way to develop gene-based inhibitors of Her2/neu over-expression or to block telomerase, which helps confer immortality on cancer cells by preventing the shortening of chromosomes associated with cell division, but widespread treatments are still in the future. There are still major stumbling blocks on how to deliver the gene to every breast cell in adults. There is also the complex ethical issue of getting the replacement gene into the germline to prevent the transmission of the defective gene to subsequent generations. In animal studies, new genes are introduced into the germline by the use of embryonic stem cells, which have the potential to form any tissue or can be integrated into a developing embryo. Current federal restrictions on the use of human embryonic stem cells will only intensify the debate and delay the potential of this avenue of research.

Focus on Prevention and Control If Not Cure

As mentioned earlier, a major current focus of breast cancer research is on prevention and control. Understanding the complex interaction of susceptibility genes and environmental stimuli including dietary factors may lead to drugs and even vaccines that may help prevent the disease in high-risk people. Further understanding of the role of epigenetic interactions, may enable control of the disease, even if a cure is not feasible.

Drugs or other preventive agents may block the effect of the carcinogen(s) that initiate the change from a normal cell to a premalignant one. Gene therapy may block the effects of the mutation caused by the carcinogen. If the mutation in the cell cannot be blocked by gene therapy, drugs may act epigenetically to keep the mutant cell in control by encouraging normal cellular differentiation. Alternatively, drugs may eliminate the mutant cell by inducing apoptosis. If the mutant cell persists, other drugs are used to arrest it by blocking DNA synthesis and cell division, and by blocking angiogenesis, necessary for adequate blood supply for the developing tumor.

Political Issues

Biomedical research is expensive, and is subject to political posturing as advocates lobby for funds for their pet diseases. Although efforts to secure funds for breast cancer research are now extremely visible, it is only in recent years that the disease entered national consciousness. As recently as forty years ago, breast cancer was considered a shameful disease, one that was kept in the closet. Patients who had suspected breast tumors signed consents for "breast surgery." If the biopsy proved to be positive, they were treated immediately with disfiguring radical mastectomies. They did not learn if they still had a breast or if they had cancer until they awoke from the anesthetic. They generally had little emotional support from their physicians or even from their families. The American Cancer Society initiated the Reach to Recovery program in 1952, in which breast cancer survivors would visit newly diagnosed (and treated) patients and reassure them that there really is life after a mastectomy. It was not until the 1970s, however, that prominent women including Betty Ford, Happy Rockefeller, and Shirley Temple Black acknowledged publicly that they had breast cancer. Their candor began to focus attention on breast cancer as a dangerous disease rather than a shameful secret. By the late 1970s women began demanding a two-step procedure in which the positive biopsy would be followed by a second surgery to remove the tumor. This gave the woman time to absorb the impact of having cancer and to consider possible treatment options. Today, the two-step procedure is routine. Over the past two decades, breast-sparing surgeries such as lumpectomies have been developed. Screening mammograms for older women have become the norm, and the benefits of early diagnosis are being appreciated.

Increased political activism and the women's liberation movement of the latter part of the twentieth century helped pave the way for increased public awareness of the need for education and funding for breast cancer. In the 1980s a number of women's groups were formed to raise more money for breast cancer research and to make mammograms more available to needy women. Among those groups was the Susan G. Komen Foundation, which sponsors the highly popular "Race for the Cure" in various cities around the country. By the 1990s, the advocacy groups were visible enough to attract Congressional attention, and funding for breast cancer research began to increase. The National Breast Cancer Coalition, a group organized in 1991 by representatives of smaller breast cancer advocacy organizations, has succeeded in obtaining increased funding from both the National Cancer Institute and from the Department of Defense. They were instrumental in developing a National Action Plan to determine where funding for breast cancer should be directed. Their current goals are to increase access and treatment to all women, including those of modest financial means. They advocate for research into the causes of breast cancer, prevention, and potential cures. As a result of their advocacy, standards are being upgraded for levels of care and more patients are being encouraged to participate in clinical trials. A variety of government agencies conduct clinical trials on new cancer treatments. These agencies include the National Cancer Institute (NCI), the National Institutes of Health (NIH), the Department of Defense (DOD), the Veterans Administration (VA), and the Food and Drug Administration (FDA). For many cancer patients, including those with breast cancer, participation in a clinical trial may offer the best treatment available.

Thanks to advocacy efforts by the National Coalition for Cancer Survivorship, the Health Care Financing Administration (HCFA), which oversees Medicare, recently began to cover the cost of routine care for cancer patients who are eligible for Medicare and who enroll in clinical trials. Although two-thirds of cancer patients are seniors and eligible for Medicare, only 3 percent enroll in these trials. In order to increase participation, HCFA is conducting education and outreach to the public.

Political awareness for breast cancer advocacy is now entering the international scene. Scientists now meet with activists and lawmakers to educate them on the basic science of breast cancer and to help them understand the need for continued support for research. The ultimate goal is to make breast cancer a preventable disease.

Other advocates are concerned about issues of genetic discrimination. Volunteer organizations such as Hadassah have mounted lobbying and educational efforts so that no person should fear discrimination for being tested for a genetic mutation.

The Role of the Media in Breast Cancer Education

Increased advocacy for breast cancer funding has led to increased media coverage of the disease. In Denver, at least one local TV station is a major supporter of the annual Race for the Cure, and encourages a buddy-check system to remind women to do monthly self-exams. Feature stories of breast cancer patients, especially survivors, appear regularly on TV and in the newspapers.

Unfortunately, the media is often motivated to report the news that sells the newspapers or increases ratings, and often sacrifices accuracy in the process. Reports of clinical studies often do not distinguish between those that are well controlled and those that are not. Observational studies may point to correlations between events or conditions, but do not determine cause and effect despite media reports to the contrary. Desperately ill patients and their families are given false hopes when the media convey promises of a new cure, only to retract the information several days later. The information is often packaged into attractive sound bites that cannot possibly tell the entire story. The Internet is now a popular source of information for breast cancer patients, but many general readers cannot determine the accuracy of this information either. Since the Internet is not regulated, it is full of hype and misinformation that can lead a patient to delay diagnosis and treatment. Professional groups such as the American Medical Writers Association advocate for responsible communication of the latest research findings and treatment recommendations. Some reliable web sites exist, but one must search to find them.

Hope for the Future

Breast cancer remains a serious illness in the early twenty-first century, but like many diseases of earlier eras it is slowly revealing its molecular secrets. The mapping of the human genome is paving the way for extensive research as to how genes work, how they are regulated, and what their protein products do in normal cells and in disease. Discoveries will lead to the development of better drugs and new methods of treatment that may ultimately prevent the disease.

The cloning of BRCA1 and BRCA2 in the past decade was a major breakthrough, but it was just a beginning in the molecular battle against breast cancer. While researchers have learned that defects in these genes (and in other cell-cycle regulators) often lead to breast and/or ovarian cancer, it has not been easy to extrapolate this knowledge to cases of sporadic breast cancer. Although we know that genetic damage is necessary for cancer to occur, BRCA1 and BRCA2 are not usually the site of damage in sporadic cases. The specific genetic damage initiating sporadic breast cancers is not yet known, nor do we yet understand the interplay between an individual's genetic constitution and possible environmental toxins. We know that both heredity and environment play a role, but the complexities of the interaction are still being deciphered. Risk factors give us probabilities but cannot totally predict whether an individual will develop the disease, or what course the disease may take. Even patients with known mutations in BRCA1 and BRCA2 are not at absolute certainty of developing cancer. It is hoped that information from the Human Genome Project will provide answers to these vexing questions of susceptibility and causation.

The ultimate research goal, to prevent breast cancer, may prove extremely difficult to achieve because the disease is so complex. We now know that the clinical expression of breast cancer is the result of multiple events that may begin years before a tumor is detected. The network of complex interactions within cells and between cells that regulate the behavior of a normal cell in a tissue ultimately determines whether a damaged cell will proliferate, remain quiescent, or die. Each cancer is unique, as is the patient bearing it.

Individuals vary not only in susceptibility to cancer but also in how they respond to drug therapy. Genes control how we metabolize certain drugs and how they are transported into cells. Drugs that work on a particular type of cancer in one patient may not be effective for another with a similar tumor. Chemotherapy doses must also be adjusted for the response of individual patients.

Advances in the Human Genome Project will most likely facilitate the design of tumor-specific and patient-specific drugs that can attack only the tumors and spare normal cells, thereby minimizing side effects. New technologies are being developed to speed the process and reduce the costs of developing these drugs. Better approaches to gene therapy are also being developed. The new DNA microarray technology already permits rapid analysis of specific patterns of gene expression in a specific tumor and may be useful in developing specific drugs that can block steps in the gene expression pathway.

While research continues into molecular strategies for arresting the disease early in its development, new conventional treatments are also being developed. Newer drugs such as Taxol and Femara are showing promise (see tables 5.3 and 5.4). Increased public awareness is helping to secure more funding for research. More women are being educated in the importance of early diagnosis and treatment. Increased political pressure is helping to secure funds for screening and, if necessary, treatment of traditionally underserved groups of women such as the medically indigent, minorities, and migrants. The war against breast cancer continues, but individual battles are being won. Better understanding of breast cancer genetics is playing a major role in these victories. It is my hope that our grandchildren will speak of breast cancer as a disease of the past.

Appendix

This appendix lists a variety of resources for people seeking information on breast cancer, cancer in general, and genetic counseling. Many of these resources provide links to other sources of information. Many helpful organizations are also listed in local telephone directories and newspaper. It may also be helpful to contact local health departments and major university medical centers if one exists in your locale.

National Programs

American Cancer Society (ACS)
Phone: 1-800-ACS-2345 (toll-free hotline for information and referrals)
Web: www.cancer.org
Sponsors "Reach to Recovery" program.

Cancer Care, Inc.
Phone: 1-800-813-HOPE
Web: www.cancercare.org
Provides support services, education, general information, referrals, and financial assistance. Published "A Helping Hand-The Resource Guide for People with Cancer" in 1997.

Hadassah-American Affairs Department
50 W. 58th Street
New York, NY 10019
Phone: 212-303-8136
Web: www.hadassah.org
Advocacy for breast cancer information and to prevent genetics-based insurance discrimination.

Living Beyond Breast Cancer
Phone: 1-888-753-LBBC (1-888-753-5222) (toll-free hotline)
Web: www.lbbc.org
A Philadelphia-based organization whose mission is to empower all women affected by breast cancer to live as long as possible with the best quality of life.

National Alliance of Breast Cancer Organizations (NABCO)
9 E. 37th Street, 10th Floor
New York, NY 10016
Phone: 1-888-80-NABCO
Web: www.nabco.org
Membership organization providing information about breast cancer.

National Breast Cancer Coalition
1707 L Street, NW
Suite 1060
Washington, DC 20036
Phone: 202-296-7477
Web: www.natlbcc.org
Coalition of cancer patients focused on changing public policy as it relates to progress against breast cancer.

National Cancer Institute (NCI)
Phone: 1-800-4-CANCER (Cancer information service)
Web: www.nci.nih.gov
Special websites include:
http://cancer.gov (general information)
http://cancertrials.nci.nih.gov (information on clinical trials)
http://cancernet.nci.nih.gov (information on cancer treat-
    ment, screening, prevention supportive care, genetics, and
    clinical trials)
For a list of NCI-designated Cancer Centers, see:
www.nci.nih.gov/cancercenters/centerslist.html

National Coalition for Cancer Survivorship (NCCS)
1010 Wayne Avenue
Silver Spring, Maryland 20910
Phone: 877-NCCS-YES
Fax: 301-565-9670
Email: info@cansearch.org
Web: www.cansearch.org
This organization supports cancer survivors and provides a helpful support service.

National Comprehensive Cancer Network (NCCN)
Phone: 1-888-909-NCCN
Web: www.nccn.org
A network of major cancer research and treatment institutions including City of Hope National Medical Center, Dana-Farber Cancer Institute, Fox Chase Cancer Center, Fred Hutchinson Cancer Research Center, H. Lee Moffitt Cancer Center and Research Institute at the University of South Florida, Huntsman Cancer Institute at the University of Utah, James Cancer Hospital and Solove Research Institute at the Ohio State University, Johns Hopkins Oncology Center, Memorial Sloan-Kettering Cancer Center; Robert H. Lurie Comprehensive Cancer Center of Northwestern University, Roswell Park Cancer Institute, Stanford Hospital and Clinics, St. Jude Children's Research Hospital, UCSF Medical Center, University of Texas M.D. Anderson Cancer Center, University of Alabama at Birmingham Comprehensive Cancer Center, University of Michigan Comprehensive Cancer Center, UNMC/Eppley Cancer Center at University of Nebraska Medical Center. NCCN experts developed the Clinical Practice Guidelines used in the Network medical centers. The Breast Cancer Treatment Guidelines for Patient, Version III, was jointly published by NCCN and ACS, June 2000.

National Society of Genetics Counselors
Web: www.nsgc.org
This is a professional organization of genetics counselors. Their website contains a link to help you find a genetics counselor near you.

Susan G. Komen Breast Cancer Foundation
Phone: 1-800-462-9273 (1-800-I'M AWARE) (Breast Care
    Helpline)
Web: http://breastcancerinfo.com
    The Foundation sponsors the Race for the Cure in many cities
each year. It supports grants for breast cancer research, and provides
lists of books and audiocassettes on such topics as breast cancer in
general, prevention, diagnosis, treatment, coping with breast cancer,
sexuality, children & family support, and numerous on-line
resources.

Y-ME National Breast Cancer Organization
212 W. Van Buren Street
Chicago, IL 60607
Phone: 1-800-221-2141 (toll-free hotline)
Web: www.y-me.org
    Provides support and counseling by trained peer counselors.
Provides hotlines for spouses of breast cancer patients and a Spanish
language hotline.

Local Programs in the Denver Area

AMC Cancer Research Center
1600 Pierce Street
Denver, CO 80214
Phone: 1-800-525-3777 (Cancer information and Counseling
    Line)
Web: www.amc.org
    Information on prevention and early detection of breast cancer

University of Colorado Cancer Center
University of Colorado Health Sciences Center
4200 E. 9th Avenue
Denver, CO 80262
Phone: 1-800-473-2288

Web: http://uch.uchsc.edu/uccc/welcome/index.html

The University of Colorado Health Sciences Center is an NCI-designated Comprehensive Cancer Center offering the latest in diagnosis and treatment at the Anschutz Cancer Pavilion on the Fitzsimons Campus. The Cancer Center includes a Hereditary Cancer Clinic.

Qualife Wellness Community
1741 Gaylord Street
Denver, CO 80206
Phone: 303-393-9355

Healing Journeys through Breast Cancer-Comprehensive support for those diagnosed with breast cancer.

International

Canadian Breast Cancer Foundation
Web: www.cbcf.org

Supports the advancement of breast cancer research, diagnosis and treatment

Canadian Cancer Society/Cancer information Service
Phone: 888-939-3333 (toll free in Canada only, English or
    French)
Web: www.cancer.ca

Hopeline
Can-Survive
Level 1, 693 Burke Road
Camberwell, Victoria
Australia
Phone: (in Australia): 1 300 36 4673 (1 300 DO HOPE)

Operating hours. Monday through Thursday from 8pm–11pm; Tuesday and Saturdays from 2pm–5pm (Melbourne time).

Hopeline is the first operational arm of the Can-Survive Hope and Survival Network, a Camberwell, Australia-based not-for-profit Public Benevolent Institution. Hopeline is the first and only telephone counseling service in the world linking patients and families facing any life-threatening illness with survivors and family members who have been through a similar crisis. Based in Melbourne, Australia, Hopeline provides emotional, spiritual, and practical support and encouragement to patients and their families in distress no matter where they live.

Notes

1. The concept of cumulative risk is often misunderstood. Because the risk of developing breast cancer increases with advancing age, the risk is additive over a lifetime. For example, for women younger than forty-nine, the risk is 2 percent (one in fifty). Between ages fifty and sixty-nine, the risk increases by 3 percent for a total of 5 percent (one in twenty). Between ages seventy and eighty-five, it increases by an additional 6 percent for a total of 11 percent (one in nine). After age eighty-five, the risk increases to 12.5 percent (one in eight), assuming the woman lives that long. Remember that these are probabilities. An individual woman could be struck with the disease at any time. If the woman carries a susceptibility gene, the probability accelerates dramatically to a lifetime cumulative risk of 56–82 percent.

2. While a mature red blood cell may never become a nerve cell, recent experiments using bone marrow stromal (lining or support) cells and stem cells (blood cell precursors) indicate that undifferentiated cells exist in the marrow that can give rise to other types of tissues if transplanted at the appropriate time. The cells may first need to be cultured with specific growth factors prior to transplantation. This exciting work gives hope for new types of therapies.

3. Dr. Susan Love (with Karen Lindsey, *Dr. Susan Love's Breast Book,* 3rd ed., Perseus, 2000) considers fibrocystic change to be a "wastebasket" of normal variations in breast tissue, rather than a pathological condition. However, atypical hyperplasia is considered to be a pre-cancerous condition that requires careful monitoring. Her bias is that, under appropriate conditions, atypical hyperplasia can be reversed and does not necessarily have to progress to cancer.

4. The term cloning is used in several different contexts:

- The process of isolating a single cell from a culture of cells, so that all subsequent progeny arise from that single cell.
- The process by which cloned animals, such as Dolly the sheep, are derived from the fusion of an adult cell (from skin or

elsewhere) and an egg cell whose nucleus has been removed. The adult cell contributes all the genetic information, and the egg cytoplasm contains the "machinery" to enable an embryo to form. Every cell in the cloned organism contains the genetic information of the adult cell.

• The process used by molecular biologists to isolate the DNA of a gene, identify it, and insert into special vectors (e.g., bacterial chromosomes) for manipulation and further study

5. This is a simplistic view to demonstrate dominant and recessive traits. Genetic control of human eye color is actually more complex and not completely understood.

6. Many genetics studies take place in Utah because the Mormon Church keeps detailed genealogical records and has done so for generations.

Glossary

Alleles Multiple forms of a gene at a given locus. Polymorphic alleles are multiple possible DNA sequences at a specific locus that are seen in at least 1 percent of the population and provide for normal variability within a species.

Angiogenesis factors Small molecules often secreted by tumor cells that cause the growth of new blood vessels to the tumor. Veg-f (vascular endothelial growth factor) is an angiogenesis factor.

Apoptosis A genetically determined "suicide" program by which a cell dies without causing a reaction that can injure surrounding tissue. Apoptosis is sometimes called "programmed cell death." The process has specific biochemical and morphological characteristics.

Aromatase inhibitors Chemotherapy drugs that inhibit aromatase, an enzyme involved in estrogen synthesis.

Atypical hyperplasia Abnormal growth of epithelial cells lining the ducts that has a high probability of progressing to cancer.

Ataxia telangiectasia (AT) A disease caused by a defective recessive gene which causes increased sensitivity to ionizing radiation and high incidence of leukemia. Homozygous women have a higher incidence of breast cancer.

Base pairing A property of the nucleotide bases of which DNA is composed. Normally, A pairs with T and C pairs with G.

Benign breast lumps These can include cysts, fibrocystic change and solid tumors called fibroadenomas. They may grow and occupy space, but are not cancer and do not invade normal tissue. Most breast lumps, especially in younger women, are benign.

BCL2 A gene expressed by cancer cells that confers protection against apoptosis and is one basis of resistance to chemotherapy.

BRCA1 and BRCA2 Tumor suppressor genes. Mutations in these genes are associated with hereditary breast cancer and some cases of ovarian cancer.

Cancer Growths or tumors composed of malignant cells that have the potential to invade normal tissues.

Carcinogen An environmental agent that causes DNA damage and cancer. Some agents cause mutations, but not necessarily cancer. Some carcinogens require assistance from other factors (promoters) to cause cancer.

Carcinoma Cancer derived from epithelial cells that line body cavities such as milk ducts.

cDNA libraries Archives of DNA segments that were copied from mRNA (c = complementary), cloned and sequenced. They are useful for identification of genes and analyses of gene expression.

Cell Basic unit of structure and function of living things. The two main compartments are the nucleus and cytoplasm. The cell is surrounded by a plasma membrane and consists of specialized molecules called proteins, lipids (fats), carbohydrates (sugars), and nucleic acids such as DNA and RNA. Genetic information is coded in DNA and stored in the nucleus. Cells are dynamic structures in which many biochemical activities occur at the same time.

Cell cycle An exquisitely controlled process by which a cell synthesizes all the necessary molecules before it divides.

Cell differentiation Process by which a cell becomes specialized to perform a specific function. As a cell differentiates, gene expression becomes limited to specific pathways, and does not revert except under extraordinary conditions.

Cell division Mechanism by which a cell proliferates. The cell copies all of its components including its genetic information, and splits into two. Two cells become four, etc. Cell division is an extremely controlled and regulated process.

centiMorgan (cM) Measure of distance between genetic markers (1 cM = 1 million base pairs of DNA).

Centromere The chromosome structure that holds the two chromatids together. The location of the centromere defines the short and long arms of the chromosome. It is also important for proper alignment of the chromatids for mitosis.

Chemoprevention Drug regimens designed to prevent breast cancer in high risk women (e.g. Tamoxifen).

Chemotherapy Treatment of a malignant tumor using toxic drugs to destroy the fast-growing cells. Chemotherapy can have severe

side effects. Often, a combination of drugs is used to help prevent the development of resistance.

Chromatid Packaging structure for DNA. Chromosomes
are seen in metaphase as two chromatids joined by the
centromere. During cell replication, chromatids separate
so that each daughter cell receives one from each
chromosome.

Chromosomes Nuclear structures that package DNA. Genes are
located at specific positions on chromosomes. Human cells contain twenty-three pairs of chromosomes.

Clonal tumors Tumors derived from a single, genetically defective cell.

Cloning This term has several distinct meanings depending upon
the context:

- The process of isolating a single cell so that all subsequent
progeny arise from this cell.
- The process by which an identical animal is created from an
adult cell.
- The process used to isolate DNA from a gene and insert it into
special vectors to manipulate it for further study.

See Reference 4 for more details.

Co-dominant alleles Each allele in a pair exerts an equal effect on
the phenotype.

Codon A sequence of three nucleotide bases (triplet) on an mRNA
molecule that corresponds to a specific amino acid. During
translation, the tRNA anti-codon binds a codon on mRNA on
the ribosome and adds the corresponding amino acid to the
growing polypeptide chain.

Connective tissue Tough, fibrous tissue that forms the framework
for tissues and organs. Collagen is the major protein of connective tissue.

DCIS Ductal carcinoma in situ. Breast cancer confined to the
ducts. DCIS may progress to invasive ductal carcinoma, the
most common type of breast cancer.

Diploid Cells containing two copies (one maternal, one paternal) of each chromosome. Normal nucleated cells, other than gametes, are diploid.

DNA (Deoxyribonucleic acid) The long, double-helical molecule that serves as a genetic blueprint for an organism. DNA is located in the nucleus and is packaged in chromosomes. Genes are composed of DNA. DNA consists of a sugar and phosphate backbone and four nucleotide bases. DNA has the ability to replicate itself by complementary base pairing.

DNA microarray (genome chip) analysis A molecular-based technology that permits rapid assessment of pathways of gene expression in normal vs. cancer cells. A sample of perhaps thousands of genes are affixed to a chip and then probed with labeled cDNA that has been expressed in cells. The probe binds to the DNA on the chip by complementary base pairing.

Dominant alleles An allele that controls the ultimate expressed phenotype.

Endometrial hyperplasia Excessive growth of the lining of the uterus (endometrium) due to excess stimulation by estrogen. This condition that may predispose to endometrial cancer. Postmenopausal women on HRT are given progesterone (or synthetic progestins) to reduce the risk of this condition.

Enzymes Specialized proteins that serve as catalysts for biochemical reactions and are necessary for the life and proper functioning of a cell.

Epigenetic events Situations in which expression of a gene is controlled by the environment surrounding the cell, rather than at the level of the gene. E.g., the stroma may prevent an early cancer in situ from becoming invasive.

Epithelial cells Cells that line body cavities, glands and surfaces including milk ducts. Cancers of epithelial cells are called carcinomas. The lining is called epithelium.

Estrogen Class of female hormones produced by the ovary and some other tissues. Estrogen plays a role in the menstrual cycle, and is important for the development of the mammary glands. Estrogen may serve as a promoter for breast cancer by stimulating cell division. Some breast cancers contain surface receptors for estrogen, which makes them more amenable to anti-estrogen therapy.

Exon Sequence of DNA that is a coding region; codes for a protein or regulatory factors.

Extracellular matrix Non-living material that surrounds cells in a tissue and plays a role in cell-to-cell communication.

Founder mutation A mutation within an isolated population that expands as the population expands.

Gamete Egg cell or sperm cell. Gametes are haploid, containing only twenty-three chromosomes.

Gene The basic unit of inheritance. Human genes consist of DNA and are located on chromosomes. Genes code for proteins in the cell.

Gene expression All genes are present in a given cell, but only certain ones function at a given time in a given cell. The others are "turned off." The genes that are "on" are being expressed, or are coding for specific proteins. Gene expression is highly regulated.

Genetic disorder Disease caused by a mutation in a gene. It may or may not be inherited.

Genetic markers Identifiable DNA sequences that serve as signposts along a chromosome which help identify the location of a particular gene.

Genome Total genetic information in the cells of a given species.

Genomics The field of study of all the genes as an integrated, dynamic system.

Genotype The alleles specific to an individual.

Germ cells Precursor cells that give rise to gametes.

Haploid Condition of cells containing only half of a normal complement of DNA. Gametes are haploid.

Her2/neu A variant growth factor receptor found on some breast cancer cells and thought to be a marker of aggressive disease.

Heterozygous Carrying two different alleles at a given locus.

Homologous chromosomes Chromosomes that are identical in loci, although alleles may differ.

Homozygous Condition in which both copies of an allele are identical.

Hormone replacement therapy (HRT) Replacement of estrogen (and for women with an intact uterus, estrogen and progesterone) to alleviate symptoms of menopause and to prevent osteoporosis.

Human Genome Project A multinational effort to map the entire human genome. Completion of a tentative map was announced by the Project and by a competing, private effort in June 2000. The discoveries and new technologies are accelerating molecular-based medicine.

Immunosuppression Weakened immune system due to drugs that destroy bone marrow. Immunosuppressed patients are at high risk for infections.

Inherited disorder A disease caused by an inherited mutation.

Intron Sequence of DNA located within a gene that does not code for its product and is removed during mRNA processing.

Invasive ductal carcinoma Carcinoma arising in the duct epithelium and invading the stroma. This is the most common breast cancer.

LCIS Lobular carcinoma in situ. This condition arises in the epithelial cells of the lobule and is considered to be a pre-malignant.

Li-Fraumeni syndrome Multiple organ cancers including breast cancer associated with inherited mutation in p53.

Linkage Association of genes based on their proximity on a chromosome.

Lobules Glandular breast tissue that synthesizes milk.

Locus Location of a gene on a chromosome.

lod score A measure of linkage between two loci (one can be a genetic marker). A lod score of three or greater indicates linkage.

Loss of heterozygosity (LOH) Loss of one of two alleles in a cell. This is a common finding in cancer cells that have become genetically unstable. Loss of normal tumor suppressor alleles is a common finding.

Lymphatic system A series of vessels that drain body tissues and carry lymph back to the circulatory system. Along the route are a series of filters called lymph nodes that trap bacteria and other "foreign invaders" and contain cells that can mount an immune response. Breast cancer cells are often trapped in lymph nodes under the armpit. Their presence indicates that the disease is spreading and can be of prognostic value.

Malignant cells Genetically altered cells that have acquired the ability to grow in uncontrolled fashion and can invade other tissues.

Malignant transformation The multi-step process by which normal cells become malignant.

Mammary gland Gland embedded in breast where, in females, milk is produced. Males have rudimentary mammary glands.

Meiosis Process of reduction division by which gametes (egg cells and sperm cells) are formed. It is similar to mitosis, except that the homologous chromosomes are delivered into sex cells. An exchange of genetic material occurs while the homologous chromosomes are next to each other, leading to a mixing of maternal and paternal genetic material.

Menarche First menstrual period. Menarche before age 12 may be a risk factor for breast cancer.

Menopause Permanent cessation of menstruation. Menopause occurring after age fifty-five may increase the risk of breast cancer. Breast cancers often behave differently if they occur before menopause (pre-menopausal) or after menopause (post-menopausal).

Metastasis Process by which malignant cells break free from the organ of origin and invade other sites in the body.

Microcalcifications A finding on mammograms of flecks of calcium in the breast. These may indicate a malignant tumor is present or may be the result of normal "wear and tear."

(Milk) ducts Conduits in the breast that carry milk from the mammary gland lobules, where it is made, to the nipple.

Mitosis Mechanism by which somatic cells divide and each daughter cell receives the same chromosome complement as the parent cell.

Multifactorial disease A disease caused by multiple genes and/or gene/environment interplay.

Multi-step carcinogenesis The mechanism by which cancers are formed by a series of sequential gene mutations, sometimes over decades.

Mutations Alterations in the normal sequence of DNA that can lead to variability but can also cause disease, including cancer. Mutations sometimes occur spontaneously, but can also be caused by toxins. Mutations in somatic cells affect the individual but are not inherited. Mutations in germ cells affect subsequent generations of offspring.

Non-coding region Sequences of DNA that do not code for proteins. They exist between genes and within them. The latter are called introns.

Nucleotide bases Four molecules that provided the coding sequences in DNA: adenine (A), thymine (T), cytosine (C), and guanine (G). They have the ability to base pair (A with T, C with G). Uracil is a nucleotide base that substitutes for T in RNA.

Oncogenes Mutated proto-oncogenes (genes that normally are involved in cell-cycle regulation, cell growth, and differentiation) that may cause a cell to proliferate out of control and lead to cancer. There are about 50–100 proto-oncogenes in humans.

Organochlorines Organic molecules bound to chlorine that are components of industrial waste that are toxic and carcinogenic. Examples include PCBs (polychlorobiphenols).

Parity Number of pregnancies.

PAX, or paired box genes Genes that are highly conserved in evolution that regulate development in many species. If mutated, they are often associated with cancer.

Perimenopause Period of time around the cessation of menstruation, during which women may experience symptoms related to decreased estrogen production.

p53 A tumor suppressor gene; controls growth-related genes. Mutations in p53 are associated with many different cancers.

Penetrance The percent of individuals carrying a gene that show the phenotype.

Phenotype The observable characteristics of an individual; the result of genes and the environment.

Polygenic disease Disease attributed by mutations in multiple genes.

Polymerase Chain Reaction (PCR) A method for amplifying sequences of DNA.

Polymorphism Variability in the DNA sequence of a gene present in 1 percent (or more) of the population. Most polymorphic alleles account for normal variability between individuals, but some are associated with disease.

Progesterone Female sex hormone produced by the corpus luteum of the ovarian follicle after ovulation. The normal role of progesterone is to prepare the lining of the uterus to receive a fertilized egg. It also plays a role in preparing the breast for lactation. The role of progesterone in breast cancer is still being studied. Synthetic progesterones are called progestins.

Proteins Molecules composed of large numbers of amino acids. Proteins provide structure to cells or enzymes, catalysts for all the biochemical reactions in a cell.

Proteomics The study of how protein products of genes are processed and modified and how they interact with other proteins and non-protein molecules.

Receptors Cell surface molecules that bind circulating hormones and other factors triggering signals that change gene expression.

Recessive alleles Alleles whose effects are seen only in the absence of dominant alleles.

Recombination Exchange of genetic material between chromosomes which normally occurs during meiosis. Recombination frequencies reveal the proximity of linked genes. The closer they are, the less likely a recombination event will occur between them.

Restriction fragment length polymorphisms (RFLPs) Random, harmless variations in DNA sequences often used as molecular markers; useful in forensics as DNA "fingerprints."

Retinoblastoma A deadly childhood cancer caused by the loss of two RB genes. The RB genes are tumor suppressor genes.

Ribosomes Structures in the cytoplasm of the cell where translation takes place.

RNA (Ribonucleic acid) RNA is a single-stranded nucleic acid composed of a sugar (ribose)—phosphate backbone, and the same four nucleotide bases found in DNA except that uracil (U) substitutes for T. RNA has several forms and functions in a cell. DNA is transcribed to messenger RNA (mRNA). Protein translation occurs on ribosomes, composed, in part, of ribosomal RNA. Transfer RNA (tRNA) brings the appropriate amino acid to the mRNA on the ribosome.

Selection A cell (or organism) with certain attributes is "selected," i.e., survives. Such a cell has a "selective advantage," whereas others are "selected against" and die.

SERMs Selective estrogen receptor modulators. These are a new class of drugs (including Tamoxifen and Raloxifene) that have estrogen effects in some tissues and anti-estrogen effects in others, depending upon the class of receptors they bind to. Soy protein is believed to be a natural SERM.

Signal transduction Cascade of molecules that convey regulatory signals from the cell surface to the nucleus to modulate gene expression.

Somatic cells Body or non-reproductive cells. Mutations that occur in these cells cannot be transmitted to the next generation but are the cause of cancer.

Stroma Scaffold-like supportive structure composed of connective tissue that provides a framework for other tissues in an organ.

Tamoxifen A SERM type of anti-estrogen often used in therapy for breast cancer, and in some cases for prevention in high-risk women.

Telomere Ends of chromosomes that shorten with each cell division, thereby conferring a finite lifespan on the cells. An enzyme called telomerase replaces the ends in cancer cells, thereby immortalizing the cells.

Tissues Units of structure and function (such as muscle or nerve) composed of a number of differentiated cell types.

Transcription The process by which the information on DNA is recorded on mRNA.

Translation The process by which the information encoded in mRNA is processed to produce a protein.

Translocation Type of mutation in which a section of a chromosome is moved to a different location on the same or another chromosome. This is a typical mutation in certain types of cancer.

Tumor heterogeneity Variability in a tumor, even if it is clonal in origin, due to genetic instability, subsequent mutations, and selection pressures.

Tumor promoters Substances that promote the effects of carcinogens by stimulating proliferation and hyperplasia in initiated cells, thereby leading to the development of cancer. Estrogen is believed to act as a promoter.

Tumor suppressor genes Genes that normally regulate cell cycle and stop proliferation. Mutations in or loss of tumor suppressor genes may lead to uncontrolled cell proliferation and cancer.

Xenoestrogens Organic chemical compounds in the environment that behave like estrogens. Xenoestrogens may cause estrogen-sensitive cells to proliferate and increase the risk for breast cancer.

Zygote Fertilized egg.

Index

Understanding Health and Sickness Series
Miriam Bloom, Ph.D., General Editor

Also in this series

Addiction*Alzheimer's Disease*Anemia*Asthma*Childhood Obesity*
Chronic Pain*Colon Cancer*Crohn Disease and Ulcerative Colitis*
Cystic Fibrosis*Dental Health*Depression*Hepatitis*Herpes*Migraine
and Other Headaches*Panic and Other Anxiety Disorders*Sickle Cell
Disease*Stuttering